Journey *to* Joyful

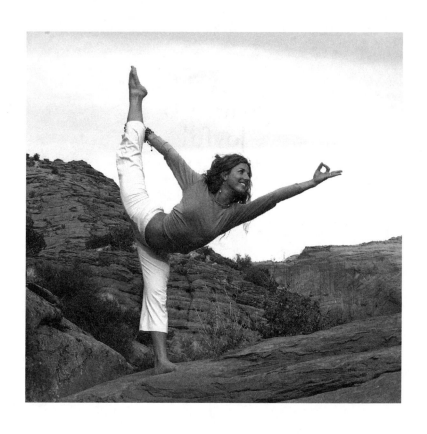

Journey *to* Joyful

Transform Your Life with Pranashama Yoga

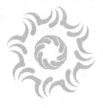

DASHAMA KONAH GORDON

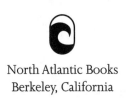

North Atlantic Books
Berkeley, California

Published by
North Atlantic Books
P.O. Box 12327
Berkeley, California 94712

Cover photo by www.starrynightphotography.net
Cover and book design by Suzanne Albertson
Illustrations on pages 8, 10, and 12 © by Sam Xavier
Photo on page 69: Wikimedia-Commons User Túrelio, Creative Commons BY-SA 2.0-de
Photo on page 92 © by audrey_sel, http://flickr.com/photos/92126232 @N00/1625782437
Photo on page 108 © Library of Congress, New York World-Telegram & Sun

Printed in the United States of America

Journey to Joyful: Transform Your Life with Pranashama Yoga is sponsored by the Society for the Study of Native Arts and Sciences, a nonprofit educational corporation whose goals are to develop an educational and cross-cultural perspective linking various scientific, social, and artistic fields; to nurture a holistic view of arts, sciences, humanities, and healing; and to publish and distribute literature on the relationship of mind, body, and nature.

North Atlantic Books' publications are available through most bookstores. For further information, visit our website at www.northatlanticbooks.com or call 800-733-3000.

Library of Congress Cataloging-in-Publication Data

Gordon, Dashama Konah.
    Journey to joyful : transform your life with pranashama yoga / Dashama Konah Gordon.
        p. cm.
    Summary: "Heartfelt personal anecdotes, easy to understand explanations of yoga philosophy, and enlivening exercises help readers to access the 'expansive openness of love within' and eliminate addiction, tame stress, enhance their well-being and sensuality, and realize their true goals in life"—Provided by publisher.
    ISBN 978-1-58394-302-1
    1. Yoga. I. Title.
RA781.7.G67 2010
613.7'046—dc22   2010042587

1 2 3 4 5 6 7 8 9   SHERIDAN   15 14 13 12 11

To all of the seekers who live courageously following their heart and dreams. You inspire the world with every thought, word, and deed. Thank you for being. To all teachers and those who have come before us to pave the way to a higher level of conscious awareness, living with love and devotion. I bow to the challenges I have faced throughout, which have led me to this present moment. I bow to the guru that dwells within us all—may we always remember to turn our eyes and ears inward to listen to the silence of our own inherent wisdom and be guided by grace.

Contents

CHAPTER 2
Navigating the Sea of Emotions 29

CHAPTER 3
Taming the Monkey Mind 75

CHAPTER 4
Spiritual Liberation 99

APPENDIX A
Self-Assessments 123

APPENDIX B
Chakras, Mantras, and the Power of Chanting 135

APPENDIX C
Organs and Corresponding Emotions 141

APPENDIX D
Introduction to the Three-Stage Energy Diet 143

A Special Thank You

This book would not be complete without the expression of my gratitude for all those who have helped me along my own Journey to Joyful.

I wish to express the deepest level of gratitude to my mother, bless her soul, who taught me yoga at a young age. She and my father also encouraged me to question everything and develop a deep sense of curiosity about life. It is through this exploration that I have come to the realization that love is the strongest power in the universe, and the highest level of enlightened bliss is accessible to us here and now in this life. Thank you, Dad, for turning your life around and being interested in healing our relationship. You reflect the kind of courage I love to see in everyone.

Thank you to Ryan Scott Seaman, the mastermind editor behind Journey to Joyful. With your creative insight and profound contribution throughout this book, I feel it will best benefit readers for years to come. And my deepest gratitude for your significant input and brilliant contribution to chapter 3, "Taming the Monkey Mind." You have the ability to transform written messages into masterpieces of poetic and intellectually stimulating imagery and art.

Thank you, Aunt Robyn, for being there for Rua and me during our time of need. Thank you for all the love you shared and the grace you demonstrated.

To my three magical, beautiful, and brilliant yoga-loving sisters who are my biggest support system and sources of encouragement. Thank you, Rua, for all the advice and for being the voice of reason to my tremendously creative spirit. Thank you, Bokhara, for all the love and light that you embody. You are such a bright light. Jophiel Angel, thank you for being such an adventurous and free-spirited example.

Thank you to all my teachers, mentors, and angels, who have been guiding me since the dawn of time. A special thank you to Amma, the embodiment of love and compassion. She is an inspiration for my life and the lives of millions globally. Shiva Rea, for being such a beautiful inspiration and courageously creative teacher; Deepak Chopra, Anthony Robbins, Jim Rohn, David Wolfe for the passion and wisdom that you share; Oprah for being one of my biggest inspirations since childhood; Sanyana Roman, Sula DePaula, and Linda Dewitt for helping me love and forgive myself and everyone, heal my heart, and embrace my inner child. Thank you, Mukti, for your brilliance, your friendship, and your profound Thai Yoga and Vedic teachings. Snatam Kaur, Wah! and all of the Bhakti Yogis who have gifted me with the blessings of *kirtan* and the healing power of *mantra*; and all the yogis, swamis, and enlightened masters who have come before us, to show us that enlightened Bliss is possible and attainable.

I also want to express my gratitude to the artists and creators of the charts and graphs included in this book. For those of you whom I was unable to contact in my attempts to receive permission to reproduce your beautiful work, I extend my humble appreciation for your creations and the immeasurable support they provide in the awakening of our collective consciousness.

Thank you Kate, Debby, Xavier, Chopp, Larisa, Scott Adams, Harlan, Sharon, Tsippy, Curtis, Eddie, Jay, Bob, and all my friends, clients, students, and fans who are so supportive and loving. I love you all. Thank you for everything!

Introduction

This book is an interactive manual designed to bring your life into balance and harmony with your highest potential. You will learn to cultivate your inner radiance and to release that which is holding you back from feeling love, joy, and success on a consistent basis. You will get back in touch with your dreams and begin to cultivate a vision for the life of your dreams. You will also learn how to actually work toward attaining that vision, step by step. I will present all of the tools, techniques, and options that you can utilize to get where you aspire to go.

While you are implementing this program, you will be manifesting positive results in all areas of your life. Through the completion of this manual, you will discover your way to living a life in harmony with the Sacred Life Force energy of the universe and continually evolving in a positive direction.

The inspiration for writing this book has come from my own path, as well as the paths of my clients, friends, and loved ones over the years. Everywhere I look, people are dealing with challenges on some level. This has been accepted as an unavoidable part of life. For many years I subscribed to this belief as well. *This all began to shift for me when I realized there are people, if only a small percentage, who live in a perpetual state of joy.* These people experience challenges like anyone else, but they handle them in a more fluid and unattached way. They don't seem to be shaken by disaster, and they learn to utilize challenges to grow even stronger and become even more grounded in the joy of living. They don't seem to be affected by the fluctuations of the economy or the changing tides of geopolitical climate. When the gas prices rise by a dollar or a winter blizzard prevents them from travelling home to be with loved ones, they are seemingly unaffected. This is the life I know I was meant to live.

This is the life we are all meant to experience.

I began studying the lives of happy, successful, and wealthy people from all walks of life, both ancient and modern. I soon learned that wealth has very little to do with financial gain and much more to do with living in balance and continual personal growth. To be affluent but unhealthy is not wealth. To be healthy with no financial freedom is not wealth. To have money and health, but to suffer emotionally and be devoid of joy is certainly not wealth. Any life lacking success and balance in any one of the five major areas—Body, Emotions, Abundance, Mind, and Spirit—will know suffering. I determined quickly that in order to get to a balanced state of being, a lot of inner reflection and healing is necessary.

Throughout this book, I refer often to my own life story as an illustration of the fact that circumstances don't have to determine the outcome of your life. Your life story can, instead, guide you, motivate you, and serve you on your path to awakening!

I was born into this world to loving parents who constantly battled with substance-abuse issues. Beginning at the age of seven, I and my three sisters bounced around from one foster home to another, until I finally found a permanent home with my aunt and uncle in the Black Hills of South Dakota. They could only house two of us, so my oldest and youngest sisters were sent off to live with relatives in Florida and New York. During those tumultuous times, I found solace in the practice of yoga.

Throughout the life lessons on my path, one of the most resounding is the depth and healing power of yoga for the mind, body, spirit, and emotions. This extends far beyond the enlivening capacity of the physical *asana* practice. The profoundly transformative value of yoga came to me through my discovery of the connection between breath and spirit, meditation, and the infinitely creative power of mental imagery. In the journaling of my experiences I discovered a canvas upon which I could attain peace by giving form to the myriad thoughts swimming through my mind.

Through a multitude of yoga practices, I experienced heart-opening sensations and true Spiritual Union. I discovered balance and harmony in my deeper appreciation that *God does not lead us through deep waters to drown us, but to cleanse us.*

When I look back at the events of my life from birth until this moment, I am immensely grateful for each and every experience. I am who I am because of them, not in spite of them. As they say, "You can't reach the highest heights without first experiencing the lowest lows." Without the presence of dark, there would be no light. Without the concept of evil, good could not exist. And the supremely sweet illumination of sunrise would never occur without the long dark night just before the dawn.

Did you know the darkest hour of night occurs just before dawn?

The construct of our universe is organized this way. Polarity exists so that we may discover the truth beyond this world of duality, which is the ultimate purpose of life according to the ancient yogis. We are born into this precious human existence to achieve the unification of opposites and become enlightened, or liberated, from the illusion of separation. This is the heart of Hatha Yoga. Ha = Sun and Tha = Moon. This time-honored practice allows us to explore and reconcile the imbalances that prevent the union of opposites and perpetuate the false sense of separation.

The key to Pranashama Yoga is to explore our practice and embrace both sides of the spectrum of life with unabashed JOY! Sometimes it's light. Other times dark. This is the nature of the waves of life force energy that we're surfing. Regardless of whether we're flying high at the peak or floating low in the valley, we have available to us the equanimity within a quiet mind and an open heart to *celebrate it all.*

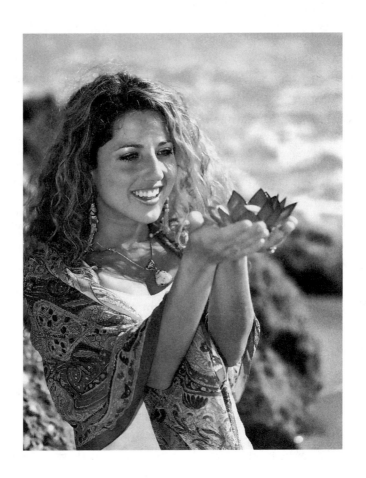

Today

I do not want to step so quickly over a beautiful line on God's
   palm
As I move through the Earth's marketplace today.
I do not want to touch any object in this world
Without my eyes testifying to the truth that everything is my
   Beloved.
Something has happened to my understanding of existence
That now makes my heart always full of wonder and kindness.
I do not want to step so quickly over this sacred place on God's
   body
That is right beneath my own foot
As I dance with precious life today.

    —Hafiz*

*Daniel Ladinsky, trans. *The Gift: Poems by Hafiz the Great Sufi Master* (New York: Penguin,
1999), 128.

CHAPTER 1

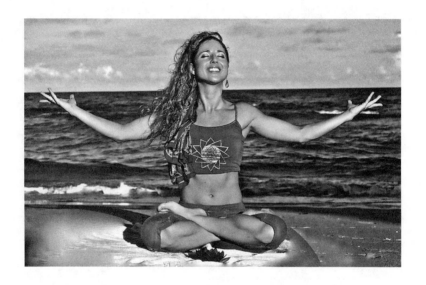

My Body Is My Temple

Yoga

Yoga: Union of the Individual self with the Universal Spirit (as in *Samadhi*).

—*Webster's Unabridged Dictionary*

Pranashama Yoga literally translates to *prana*: sacred life force energy and *shama*: calming of the mind. Thus: Sacred life force energy that calms the mind and creates union with all of existence.

P ranashama Yoga is a combination of arts including various styles of yoga (Prana Vinyasa, Ashtanga, Kundalini, Anusara, and Power styles), martial arts (T'ai Chi, Qi Gong), and Thai Yoga Therapy. This practice is designed to take you on a journey of self-discovery through your mind, body, spirit, and emotions. You will touch yourself in places you may have never known existed. You will begin to see where you have been holding and storing tension in your body; and through a process of letting go, you will begin to witness complete transformation on all levels. Once you realize how everything is interconnected, you will become very clear about what steps are necessary to raise you up to the next level in all areas of your existence.

As you may already know, yoga is a very profound path. Since it was developed more than five thousand years ago, many enlightened masters have collaborated to perfect this ancient scientific system. It encompasses every aspect of life from birth to death, explaining the soul's journey even beyond this physical realm. Within the path of yoga, there are many styles that one may gravitate toward. As you explore the hidden dimensions of who you are, you will begin to feel more in alignment with certain teachings and teachers who will guide you on your path.

Ten Golden Rules of Pranashama Yoga

Rule #1: Non-Judgment of Yourself and Others

Rule #2: Non-Attachment to Things, People, Ideas, Outcomes, etc.

Rule #3: Non-Violence to Self or Others (this includes animals, Mother Earth, etc.)

Rule #4: Never Make Assumptions

Rule #5: Be Grateful—Your Life Is a Miracle

Rule #6: Be Generous with Your Kindness, Compassion, and Forgiveness

Rule #7: Breathe Through the Pain, It Always Gets Easier with Time

Rule #8: Take Care of Yourself First—It's Easier to Serve Others That Way

Rule #9: Be Open to All Possibilities; Move Beyond the Duality of Right and Wrong

Rule #10: Always Do Your BEST, Give Your ALL, and Choose Love in Each Moment

My Body Is My Temple

The body is the most tangible aspect of who we are. It is visible and can be touched. Many people are so enthralled with the physical aspect of their being, they actually forget that the body is just one layer to the multidimensional beings that we are. On the other hand, sometimes life gets in the way, and the physical body can be completely ignored as we place priority upon other areas of our existence.

After researching and exploring just about every school of thought, I have come to understand that the ancient science of yoga offers the most complete mind, body, and spirit education available in the world. Many schools have a profound understanding about one or two of these life components, but I find that yoga offers the most encompassing approach to our human existence. The Vedic system provides a thorough understanding of the gross, subtle, and causal dimensions of life in this world. The ultimate goal of this system is to attain "enlightenment" and complete Union with the Supreme Source. This ultimately is the *Journey to Joyful* and the primary reason I am so passionate about sharing this gift with the world. Through Pranashama Yoga you will learn things about yourself that you may have never imagined.

Since yoga originated in India more than five thousand years ago, many of the terms used to describe the philosophy and physical practice come from the Sanskrit language. Throughout this book, I offer both the Sanskrit and English translation for many concepts, in an effort to keep it simple while maintaining the integrity of the lineage and origin. Additionally, I refer to "God" by many different names: the Supreme Source, the Divine, God, Creator, Creative Source of all life, and so on. All are referring to the same ineffable divinity, and I will do the best I can to honor that which transcends the very concept of words while conveying these messages as clearly as I can.

Getting to Know Your Body

In this section, you will learn about the multi-layered anatomy of yoga. Beyond the physical body, we'll explore all the energy centers and keys necessary to a complete understanding of your own body. This will enable you to grasp the concepts in later sections of this book with a strong foundation, and this section can provide a point of reference to return to throughout.

The Seven Chakras and Your Energy Centers

If you are uncertain whether we have a spirit, or soul, in this bag of bones called the human body, allow the following information to illuminate such a reality. Five thousand-plus years of wisdom and personal accounts from yogic masters, in addition to the work of the scientific and psychological communities, offer validation and support for the realization of this inner Self.

> **Chakra** is the Sanskrit term used to describe the various energy vortices positioned on the body. Each corresponds to a major aspect of your character, as well as to a color that carries a very specific frequency.

Scientific Elaboration

Frequency is the term used to measure the number of periodic oscillations, vibrations, or waves per unit of time. We are composed of millions of atoms and molecules vibrating at various frequencies. Within each atom and molecule in the universe are protons, neutrons, and electrons. The majority, more than 90 percent, of the universe is simply empty space, also referred to as the Void. It is in the open space of the Void that we experience peace, clarity, and divine intuition. This is also where we can enter into a unified state with the Supreme Source (a state called *Samadhi*) while in meditation. This will be explained in further detail in Chapters 3 and 4.

We know from physics and the laws of nature that the color with the lowest frequency on the spectrum is red, and it parallels the first chakra (root/*Muladhara*).

Moving up in frequency and running parallel with the colors of the rainbow, the next octave is orange and represents the second chakra (sacral/*Svadhisthana*).

The third chakra (solar plexus/*Manipura*) is connected to the color yellow.

Green is the color and frequency of the fourth chakra (heart/*Anahata*).

Blue corresponds to the fifth chakra (throat/*Vishuddha*).

Indigo is the color that parallels the sixth chakra (mind/third eye/*Ajna*).

The seventh chakra (crown/*Sahasrara*) is associated with the colors purple, gold, and white. This final octave is connected to the Divine or Angelic frequency through the crown of our head.

There are many books available that delve deeper into the specifics of the chakra system and how you can use it to heal and balance your life. The present book provides the fundamentals of this science, including how to apply specific techniques to unblock, balance, and enhance your chakras.

The following images offer a visual for the seven-chakra system, which is currently the most commonly used of all the systems known at this time. I believe that an understanding of these models can provide a deeper exploration into the vastly mysterious realms of human consciousness and potential. As we progress forward in our quest for conscious human evolution, we can use the discoveries of the ancient yogis to help illuminate the path. I am honored to share with you the truth of what I have come to know. (See Appendix B for more detailed descriptions of each chakra.)

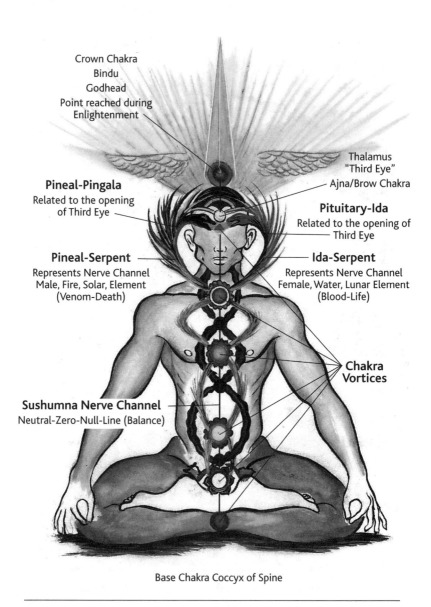

Crown Chakra
Bindu
Godhead
Point reached during
Enlightenment

Thalamus
"Third Eye"
Ajna/Brow Chakra

Pineal-Pingala
Related to the opening
of Third Eye

Pituitary-Ida
Related to the opening of
Third Eye

Pineal-Serpent
Represents Nerve Channel
Male, Fire, Solar, Element
(Venom-Death)

Ida-Serpent
Represents Nerve Channel
Female, Water, Lunar Element
(Blood-Life)

**Chakra
Vortices**

Sushumna Nerve Channel
Neutral-Zero-Null-Line (Balance)

Base Chakra Coccyx of Spine

The human body and the seven major energy centers, with the energy lines or
nadis connecting them.

Five Bodies (*Koshas*)

We spend most of our lives learning about the physical body, because that is the most tangible aspect through which we see, feel, touch, taste, and smell. The ancient yogis revealed to us the presence of five bodies, four of which exist beyond the physical realm, but all of which influence and are influenced by our experience in the human body.

Beyond the physical body that we see in the mirror are the following "layers" of our spirit. With the understanding of these layers, or *koshas*, we can begin to see how the practices and techniques of the Pranashama Yoga system can help to transform your life.

First body (*Annamaya kosha*) corresponds with the **physical** realm.

Second body, or the first layer beyond the physical body, is called *Pranamaya kosha* and corresponds with **energy** (*prana*). This layer houses the chakras.

Third body (*Manomaya kosha*) is the layer of your spirit that corresponds with **emotions** and thought patterns.

Fourth body (*Vijnanamaya kosha*) is the layer of your spirit that correlates with intuition, **wisdom,** and visionary creativity.

Fifth body (*Anandamaya kosha*) is the layer of your spirit that correlates with **Bliss,** the connection to our natural Self that is completely whole and unified with the Supreme Source. I like to call it "the Bliss channel"!

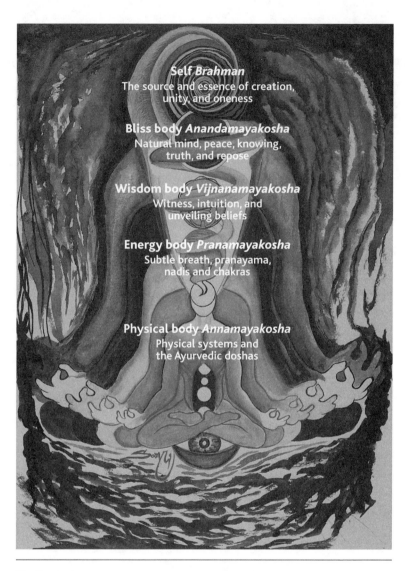

Self *Brahman*
The source and essence of creation, unity, and oneness

Bliss body *Anandamayakosha*
Natural mind, peace, knowing, truth, and repose

Wisdom body *Vijnanamayakosha*
Witness, intuition, and unveiling beliefs

Energy body *Pranamayakosha*
Subtle breath, pranayama, nadis and chakras

Physical body *Annamayakosha*
Physical systems and the Ayurvedic doshas

The Five Koshas

The Spine

Grasping the importance of your spine is essential to an understanding of your body. The spine is the support structure and is directly linked to six of the seven chakras on the body.

The yogic concept of the *sushumna* involves a central energy channel that aligns with the spine perfectly, originating at the base of the spine (sacrum) and traveling through the top bone (Mouth of God) positioned at the very top of the cervical spine, scientifically known as the atlas. It is a channel through which *prana* (spiritual energy or life force) can flow and circulate freely when unobstructed.

The two "serpents" that are winding up the spine of the man depicted in the figure on page 10 are referred to as *Ida* and *Pingala*. These represent our *Ida*/feminine (passive) and *Pingala*/masculine (active) aspects. This imagery is also known to represent lunar and solar, receptive and assertive, and so forth,

According to the teachings of ancient yoga masters as well as intuitive healers, the condition of the physical body is directly reflective of the psychosomatic (mental/emotional) condition and what the soul is communicating to the individual about his or her evolutionary journey. On the physical level, each section of the spinal column also corresponds to a bodily organ.

It is interesting and important to know that the physical concerns and misalignment we experience in the spinal vertebrae are often directly correlated with the spiritual energetic ability to flow freely.

Body Functions and the Autonomic Nervous System

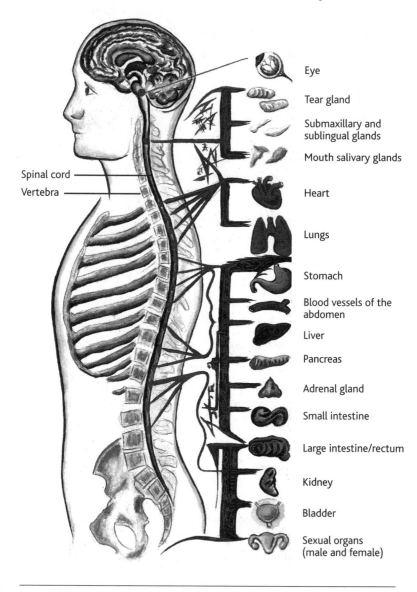

Eye

Tear gland

Submaxillary and sublingual glands

Mouth salivary glands

Heart

Lungs

Stomach

Blood vessels of the abdomen

Liver

Pancreas

Adrenal gland

Small intestine

Large intestine/rectum

Kidney

Bladder

Sexual organs (male and female)

Spinal cord

Vertebra

Functions of the body and the autonomic nervous system.

A personal example: When I first moved to Florida in 2000, I was hit by a car while riding my bicycle across a major intersection of a four-lane highway in the rain. The car that hit me was driving over 40 mph. My bike chain skipped a link and I couldn't move forward. In the split second I had to think, I believed the speeding cars would need to slow down for the red light anyway. I was shocked when an approaching car didn't slow down and smashed into my bike, catapulting me fifteen to twenty feet across the rain-soaked asphalt road upon which I painfully landed.

After a few hours in the emergency room, and despite the doctor's advice to get additional therapeutic care, I insisted that I was fine and wanted to be released immediately. Little did I know that my stubbornness would later bring me a great deal of pain.

In 2006 I began to develop discomfort and tension in my upper back and neck. By 2007 I was in need of massage therapy on a weekly basis. My condition worsened and could have been completely debilitating if not for the saving graces of my yoga, self-massage, and spiritual practices. A chiropractor informed me that I was operating with only 30 percent of my capacity (mentally and physically), and while it was disconcerting to know that my energy was so limited, I was also inspired. I felt like I was doing pretty good as I was, but the thought of such a great increase in capacity was very promising.

After a full year of treatment along with a daily yoga practice and refining my diet considerably, I felt dramatically better. I had such a reduction in my bodily tension and stress that I found yet another level of gratitude for the immeasurable healing power and beauty of yoga. Allergies that once plagued me have vanished, and my enjoyment of all areas of my life—and especially my yoga practice—has grown exponentially! I can do arm balances and head stands without causing painful after-effects, and I am excited to see what the future brings as my spine continues to restore itself back to its perfect alignment.

The relief I feel on the emotional, mental, and spiritual levels is significant as well. As you learned from the information about the five *koshas*, all bodies are influenced when we affect one of them. It was this experience, among others, that inspired me to create the 30-Day Yoga Challenge. Someone once said, "A blessing is only a blessing when you share it with other people." It has become one of my greatest joys to share the life-enhancing gift of a daily yoga practice, the benefits of a holistic approach to healthy eating, and a renewed passion for living.

Cultivating Radiance

One goal of this program is to cultivate radiance, defined as the quality of being bright and sending out rays of light. This manifests as an attractive combination of good health and happiness; "the radiance of her countenance." Good health is the state of being vigorous and free from bodily or mental disease. Happiness, felicity—such a state of well-being is characterized by emotions ranging from contentment to intense joy.

There are several key lifestyle components essential to cultivating radiance.

You Are What You Eat

When we mindlessly eat whatever fast food we can find, we see the negative effects very plainly. We see those French fries on our thighs. The ice cream sundae with hot fudge hangs out on the hips. That lower belly bulge that won't go away, regardless of how many sit-ups you do, is in all likelihood the result of the margaritas and nachos you consumed Friday night. More important than the aesthetic impact is the negative impact on our body's intestinal tract and other organ functions. Our bodies have to expend a great deal of energy to process these toxins. Even if you are not eating these types of foods on a regular basis, you will see them on your body and they will clog your organs in more ways than the FDA should ever allow.

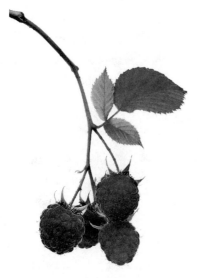

When you become more conscious of what you are putting into your temple, you will start to see your body transform, and you will be amazed at the radiant beauty hiding beneath the extra pounds. The energy you free up when you clear "non-nutritional" food from your system and nourish your body properly will serve to enhance your radiance and attractiveness exponentially. Please refer to the Three-Stage Energy Diet section in Appendix D of this book for more information about what to consume to maximize your health and radiance. The full Three-Stage Energy Diet program is detailed at www.30dayyoga challenge.com.

You Are What You Think

If you spend your day constantly thinking about how out of shape you are or feel, you progressively become more out of shape. Conversely, if you hold the *mantra* in your mind that you are continually becoming more healthy and radiant, that is what you will become. Thoughts are one of the most creative powers we have as human beings. In fact, it could be said that "What we think about we bring about."

What are your current beliefs about your physical body? Do you give thanks daily for the optimal functioning of your body, this miraculous machine created by the Divine Source? These thoughts will be reflected in your presence, health, and happiness. When we carry thoughts of negativity and self-criticism, we inspire and feed energy to precisely what we *don't* want: poor health and an unattractive physical body. Some of the best practices to reverse negative thought forms include working with affirmations, chanting *mantras*, singing, and meditation. All of these will be discussed in more detail in Chapter 3, "Taming the Monkey Mind." For now, let it suffice to say that this is an aspect of your daily habitual programming that will need to be "cleaned up" in order for you to maximize your radiance.

Your Body Is a Map of Your Past

Your body is a physical representation of the cumulative effect of all the experiences you've had throughout your life. There is a wonderful book called *Hidden Messages in the Body*, which details specifically the emotional, spiritual, and mental links to any physical ailment. These subtle levels exist in the bio-energetic field surrounding one's physical body. If you release a trauma on one level, you will experience relief on all levels. An example: let's say you tend to carry tension in your hamstrings and in your hips. This corresponds to your first and second chakras, which represent your ability to feel grounded and your freedom to flow.

Often when these chakras are blocked by unreleased trauma, it can be difficult to feel rooted in your community and more difficult still to find your natural flow wherever you live. Also in this chakra your financial, emotional, and sexual energy are reflected. If your hips are tight, it's possible that you need to release an emotional trauma that occurred in your sexual history, or in the process of giving birth to a child. This can also relate all the way back to childhood and how your parents' relationship to the physical realm was modeled for you. Children can't help but internalize their parents' beliefs without realizing it and later manifest health issues that can be linked to their belief systems about sex, money and/or their body.

The good news is once you have the map of your body, it is very clear which areas you need to work on. A tight upper back and shoulders or a tendency to chronically get injured can mean a weakness or contraction in the heart chakra. Chronic neck and upper back pain and tension can indicate that you feel the weight of the world on your shoulders, and you need to openly and honestly communicate that you need help. When we are open, strong, and fluid in our body, we are experiencing the best that life has to offer with very little limitation or constraint.

Your Body Is *Sacred*

I know a lot of people who treat their body as a temple. This beautiful home to your soul is the only one you get, so it is imperative that you take care of it. On the other hand, I've seen a lot of people who neglected their bodies and are now suffering excruciating pain that could have been avoided. You first have to decide how you want to live and feel. If you desire to live pain-free and healthfully, follow the 30-Day Yoga Challenge program. It emphasizes treating yourself with the highest love and best care at all times. In every moment we are faced with choices that will serve our highest intentions, or gratify our unconscious desires.

As an example of this, let's say you are deciding what to eat for lunch. You're selecting from a hamburger or a chicken sandwich with cheese, bacon, and mayo on a white roll with your favorite Cajun curly

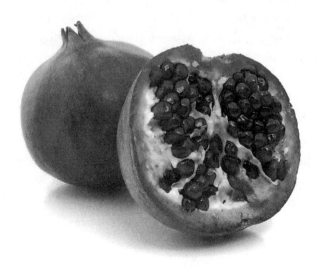

fries. The other option is a healthy salad with raw pumpkin seeds and hemp seeds with a light vinaigrette. The obvious health choice is the salad, but why do so many people choose the other? Inherent in our culture is the idea that a salad is deprivation, and a "hearty meal" or "comfort food" is fulfilling. It's ironic, really. You will feel much more fulfilled and "comfortable" when your body gets the nutrients it needs to thrive, as opposed to forcing yourself to process starches and toxins that offer little to no nutritional benefit.

Your Body Needs Rest

Sleep is an undeniably essential aspect of life, yet it is overwhelmingly misunderstood. Why do some people need more sleep than others? Why do you sometimes still feel tired when you wake in the morning? I have been told that when we harbor a lot of repressed trauma in our subconscious mind, it drains our *prana*, or life force energy. This means that we are trying to figure out how to heal while we sleep and it takes more time and energy. This can also interrupt our sleeping patterns and cause us to get restless sleep. This is a common ailment. Repressed sadness and pain from childhood or even later in life results in the heavy head syndrome. Sleep difficulties are compounded when people spend the crucial evening hours in front of the TV, where our energy is unable to relax, and when they eat too late, overburdening the digestive system while they sleep.

When we change our habits, we can change our life experience.

Try going to sleep earlier. Don't watch TV after 8 p.m. Don't eat after 8 p.m. either. Wind down for the evening with a warm bath, candle light, and relaxing music. Your internal rhythm will thank you. You will wake in the morning revived and refreshed, possibly better than you have felt in years.

Is there anything you can do to feel more alive instead of consuming caffeinated or other "energy-enhancing" beverages?

All of the prana-enhancing recommendations in this book will help. Yoga, T'ai Chi, qi gong, Reiki, pranayama, consuming fresh organic raw or living foods, drinking plenty of water, dancing, exercising, and spending time in communion with nature will all help.

Stop right now and notice how you are breathing. Are you breathing deeply? Into your belly? Filling your lungs completely? Sitting up straight so the energy can travel along the central channel (sushumna) of your spine, from the base to the crown of your head and back down? This little technique of sitting up straight and breathing deeply will dramatically change your energetic experience in life. Try it for a week, and see for yourself!

Play Like a Kid and Have Fun!

For some reason many adults stop playing as they age. It's as if they feel that playing is for kids and they can't subscribe to that mentality anymore. This is ludicrous. We choose our reality. We get to decide what we want to do with our time and our lives. An important part of being in your body is using it to do the things you enjoy. That can include playing, dancing, singing, running, jumping, skipping, swimming, and anything that reminds us of our freedom to play!

A great way to tap into your inner child is to be around children. Pay attention to their free-flowing energy and take a moment to see life through their eyes.

Children are a perfect example of how to follow your energy, play when you want to, and rest when you need to. Remember when you were a kid and you took naps? This is something I highly recommend in moments when life affords this luxury. This life is about honoring your natural rhythm and taking care of your self first. When you try to be the most vital version of your self, you can better take care of those you love.

What do you see when you look in the mirror?

This is so interesting. Most people see something entirely different than what other people see. What we see from our own eyes is clouded with false perceptions like judgment and rejection. We look around and compare ourselves to others and then come back and criticize areas where we think we don't "measure up." This is a huge schism in our psyche and something that affects us on all levels—emotionally, mentally, spiritually, and physically. You have to begin to see yourself as the perfect creation that you are. But at the same time, recognize with sincere honesty the areas that are out of balance.

Sometimes we are so blinded to reality, we no longer see ourselves anymore. This happened to a client of mine. He told me that he had been looking in the mirror and didn't see he was overweight for more than a decade. (He was carrying an extra 80 pounds!) It wasn't until he was at the beach people-watching and saw an obese man in a Speedo with his belly protruding that the light suddenly switched on and he realized, "That is me!"

Wow! This awareness takes humility, courage, and self-love. That is why it often takes so long to make a change. Our ego won't allow us to admit that we have been blind this whole time. But when you are finally ready—when enough is enough—you will know. Then the veil of illusion (*maya* in Sanskrit) will lift for you, and you will be ready to do whatever it takes to regain wholeness.

The path to wholeness is the journey to self-love.

It is such a sweet and beautiful journey, full of challenges and blessings. Welcome it all with an open heart and mind, and you will enjoy the process. On the other hand, if you attempt to travel the path with contempt and resistance to growth and change, you will struggle and not enjoy it. The choice is yours!

**Love is always there waiting to hold your hand
and lead you with grace.**

Sexuality, Sensuality, and the Physical Body

As a student and practitioner of Tantra Yoga, I feel strongly about allowing this body to be a vessel for pleasure. Why not? Many religions and other belief systems place unnecessary limitations upon what we should be "allowed" to experience, and it makes no sense to me that a God is sitting up in the sky and judging us for experiencing pleasure. It is certainly nothing to be ashamed of or to feel guilt for. I have explored both ends of this spectrum, from total celibacy to unadulterated pleasure-seeking, and found my way back to the center again. I believe, as sensory beings, we are capable of experiencing divine union with our beloved through this human body. In this sacred dance it is essential to acknowledge and honor the spirit within each body, and all other aspects of the subtle and causal energies we have access to. This takes time and is certainly a path to study and respect. To speak of the physical body in regard to sexuality, though, is key to bringing balance into our lives.

First we must feel safe and free within ourselves. If we are self-critical and feeling unworthy, it will be reflected in our sexual and intimate interactions with a partner. This can cause inhibition, contention, and dissatisfaction. Also, you will notice that the negative emotions that arise for you before, during, and after sexual experiences are always signals to look deeper within YOU. It is rarely your partner's "fault" or issue that is causing your angst. It is you. The sooner you humbly acknowledge these "inner demons" or dis-eases in your pain body, the sooner you will be on your way to wholeness, opening to your natural state of joy and bliss.

Your Body Was Created to MOVE

With the rate of obesity in the U.S. growing in both adults and children, it appears evident that people are lazy. We cannot avoid the sad truth that our lifestyles seem to avoid regular physical movement. In addition, the horrendously poor nutrition in this country affects both energy level and body functions. A television and a bag of chips will all too often trump an evening walk and a bottle of water.

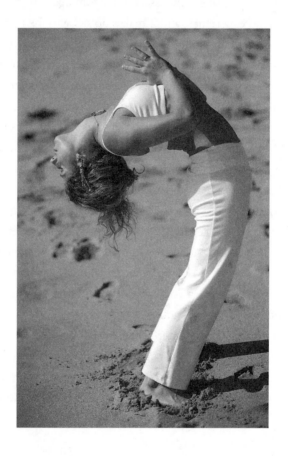

Movement should be joyful!

We are designed to process and move energy through our bodies, and we have a plethora of choices when it comes to exercise. Exercise is sometimes perceived as painful or like "work." Exercise sounds and looks so much like the word "Exorcise"! Although to a certain extent they are similar: both eradicate the toxins and negative energy from our systems and free us from static lethargy and pain. It all depends upon what movement activities you participate in.

It is time we gave the process of movement a new name—one that would inspire and motivate you simply by hearing or thinking the word! Perhaps "Dance" or "Play" should be considered.

I strongly recommend to my clients that they find hobbies that are active and fun for them. That way it doesn't have to be a scheduled allotment of time in the gym pumping iron and running on a treadmill. It can be something you look forward to. Something that you just can't wait to do. And at the same time, it is healing you, uplifting and rejuvenating, while strengthening you in more ways than you realize.

Some of my favorite methods of movement include: yoga, dancing, swimming, hula hooping, hiking, kick boxing, rock climbing, playing games like soccer and volleyball, and sports like kite boarding, surfing, and paddleboarding.

Do whatever inspires you!

If you don't have anything that fits that description yet, try taking some classes or lessons and see what you enjoy most. The important part is that you begin. And you do it because you see the value and truly want to move your body and maximize your human potential.

Finding a friend or partner who can participate with you is a wonderful way to stay motivated. When you have an accountability partner, you are much more likely to succeed and stick with your new endeavors. On the other hand, don't be discouraged if you don't have anyone.

Join a class or a club or similar group and you will meet others just like you. Then you may get an added bonus and make some new friends!

Pranashama Yoga *Asanas*

Pranashama Yoga includes a complete system for physical movement. Physical yoga poses, traditionally known as *asanas*, are designed to free our mind and body from tension and stress. They relax, rejuvenate, balance, strengthen, and energize, bringing the body and the mind into a harmonious union. *Asanas* should be done with comfort, ease, alertness, and steadiness, achieving a balance between ease and effort.

Is Yoga Spiritual or Physical?

In the West the appearance of the physical body is highly regarded. So it is not surprising that we have taken that aspect of the yoga practice and made it into the primary focus. Discussions are now under way about whether it is an athletic sport that should be included in the Olympic competitions. I support both sides of the conversation. On one hand, I know that yoga is a system designed to unify the practitioner with the Supreme Source. In this way it is absolutely a spiritual practice. The *asana* practice (physical practice of yoga) is the most popular and recognizable aspect of this ancient system. In fact, the *asana* practice was developed to get the body in the best physical condition possible, so that the yoga practitioner would be able to sit for many hours comfortably in meditation. In order to reach the higher spiritual vibrations we must be as strong, flexible, and open as possible. Why? If we are not living in our bodies, honoring them as our temple, we are closing off the divine channels (*nadis*) of energy that run through us. Additionally, when we are not in good physical shape, we limit our enjoyment of our life experience. Thus, yoga is spiritual *and* physical.

It's All Yoga

Being a lifelong athlete and fitness enthusiast, I have enjoyed almost every form of movement available on Earth. I have come full circle and believe yoga to be the most comprehensive system for human evolution of mind, body, spirit, and emotions.

When you grasp the yogic principles and philosophies, you can apply them to any activity you are doing. Then everything you do is spiritually enhancing your life. And this leads to the ultimate experience where everything you do is yoga. It is all Union, unifying you with the Supreme Source. Whether you are walking the dog, ice skating in the park, or climbing up the side of a rock cliff, when you are mindful of Spirit and connecting to the breath with an open heart, it's yoga.

The Power of *Asana* Practice

The *asana* practice is extremely powerful and unique in design. In addition to improved flexibility, circulation, muscular strength, and increased energy, as well as detoxification of the organs, each pose unblocks life force energy or *prana* pathways in your body, reprograms your cellular DNA, and connects you to your spiritual origin.

A little knowledge of Sanskrit, the ancient Indian language through which the practice of yoga was created, informs us that many of the advanced yoga *asanas* are named after Hindu gods, saints, and enlightened masters. When we practice these *asanas*, we are honoring and invoking the spirit of the master during our practice. Please don't worry that yoga will contradict your religious belief system, as Pranashama Yoga embraces all religions and belief systems. I believe we are all One and that Love is the highest truth. Love is my religion. This topic is elaborated upon in Chapter 4 of this book, "Spiritual Liberation," where I dive deeper into the all-embracing spiritual teachings of the Pranashama Yoga system.

If you currently believe in a more monotheistic approach to spirituality, some of these teachings may feel foreign to you. Please maintain an open mind while exploring the depth and wealth of wisdom that is available through the practice of yoga. You may soon come to see the union of all religions and philosophies if you maintain an open mind and heart. Maintaining an ongoing practice has been psychologically proven to create strong neuro-patterns as we bridge the gap between the conscious and unconscious mind. This serves to instill a long healthy relationship with the practice of yoga and your embrace of a new holistic lifestyle.

This book is primarily an introduction to the Pranashama Yoga method and philosophy. Future books and training manuals will more elaborately illustrate specific *asana* sequences and protocols. You can also learn more deeply about the specific *asana* sequences, *pranayama* practices (breathing exercises), and guided meditations through the yoga DVDs, videos, and audio programs available, as well as attending our workshops, trainings, and retreats held around the world. See Appendix G for information about workshops, and please visit the Pranashama Yoga website (www.dashama.com) to see a current calendar of events.

See Appendix E of this book for full descriptions of the Eight Limbs of Yoga, as detailed by Patañjali, the grandfather of modern-day yoga. This is one of the foundations of the Pranashama Yoga system, which is based upon the wisdom of the ancient yogic masters.

A True Transformation Story: The Healing Power of Yoga

by Melanie Younger, Ottawa, Ontario

Namaste.

My name is Melanie. When I was twenty-two, I found myself post-graduation in an unhealthy job, an unhealthy relationship, and thoroughly unhealthy and unhappy on all levels. In fact, I had created my life with such unhealthy patterns that my body decided to just check out. I hit rock bottom when I developed severe pneumonia in both lungs.

I spent three months taking many trips to the doctor, getting several chest x-rays, and consuming round after round of stronger and stronger antibiotics. Nothing would give. It was as though my body was having a stand-off with my mind, my life, and the choices I had made with the sacred yet uncovered parts of myself. I spent most of those three months confined to my bed, lungs so swollen and unhappy that they rubbed against my ribs with each breath. It became clear to me that if something didn't change quickly, I would likely die from this break-down of my body.

Fortunately, my mother had a friend who is a beautiful and amazing alternative healer. After one trip to her for some acupuncture, Reiki, and kind guidance for my soul, the infection moved from both of my lungs to my ear. Within seventy-two hours I was almost completely back to normal—only now I had a new perspective and increased reverence for having truly experienced gratitude for every breath.

After spending three months in bed struggling to breathe, things I had previously taken for granted became challenges. My physical body had been weakened and my lungs needed rehabilitating. It dawned on me that I had become distanced from the yoga practice my mother taught me when I was young. I made a trip to the bookstore and found an introductory yoga DVD. This became my touchstone.

Yoga was exactly what I needed to find my way back into a deep and loving relationship with my body. After struggling so hard for so long to simply inhale a full belly breath, it became a delicious luxury to breathe long, slow, and steady breaths. My tired body found a soft place to land in the *asana* practice, and learning more about my body helped me to make the necessary lifestyle choices to come into a greater place of contentment and peace with myself.

In yoga we recognize that our physical challenges, including illness, can be our greatest teachers. I benefited from the "tough love" school that the universe presented me when I needed it the most. Sometimes when you learn the hard way, your life becomes full of soft places to land, so much so that you learn to be one for others. That is my hope for my presence in the world now.

My experience with illness, alternative healing, and yoga truly changed my life and now there's no looking back (and no looking forward). There's just here and now with the breath and an unwavering belief in the light that lives in you and in me. Sometimes our body brings us a call to action. For me that call was to find a way to get to know my body, to learn to listen to it, and to love it the best way possible. For me the path and the destination are yoga.

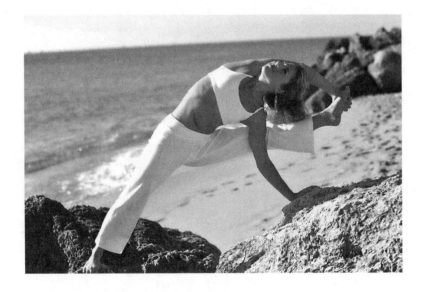

CHAPTER 2

Navigating the
Sea of Emotions

An *emotion* is a mental and physiological state associated with a wide variety of feelings, thoughts, and behavior. Emotions are subjective experiences, or experienced from an individual point of view. Emotion is often associated with mood, temperament, personality, and disposition.

—*Wikipedia*, 2009

I spent most of my lifetime in a tumultuous sea of emotions. Born in the center of the most emotionally sensitive sign in astrology, Cancer/July month, I have experienced every possible variation of emotion that exists. When I was younger this was very challenging. For most of my life, I didn't understand why I felt everything so deeply. On the other hand, it helped me to connect with a tremendous variety of people, as I have been able to relate to and empathize with almost every possible permutation of emotion that may exist in the universe. For this reason, I have also attracted students and clients for years with a wide variety of emotional issues that we've been able to work through together.

A wise man learns from his own mistakes.
An enlightened man learns from the mistakes of others.

—Zen Proverb

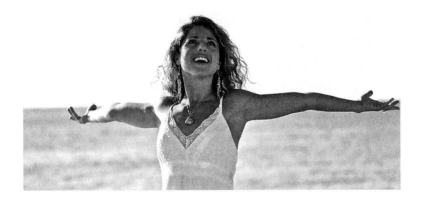

In the endless sea of emotions we all go through, I suggest you act from a place of enlightenment from here on out. I'm not suggesting that you not *feel* your emotions, quite the contrary. Feel whatever arises fully, and then let it go. I'm inviting you to let go of any *identification* with what you're feeling. You are at choice. You don't have to go through another moment of suffering. Break free from the societal constructs that say, "Life is meant to be a challenge." This is not exactly true. You have the capacity to become the observer of your emotional reactions and to check in with your heart each time, to respond from love and compassion. This is the key to becoming liberated from the bonds of emotional suffering.

In Buddhism there is a *mantra, Om mani padme hum,* which carries the vibration of compassion. This is compassion for oneself and for others. Loosely translated, it means *the jewel is in the lotus.* In other words, inside your heart lives the non-dual current of unconditional love.

Five Steps to Gain Control of Your Emotional Body

1. **Breathing is #1.** Stop and take ten deep breaths into your heart center. Practice *pranayama* (conscious breathing techniques designed to clear the pranic body or *pranamaya kosha*) to help with your emotions. This is explained in greater detail later in this chapter.

2. **Ask yourself:** What is the root of this emotional stirring?

3. **Ask yourself:** What is my vision for the best possible outcome for this situation?

4. **Ask yourself:** If God were watching my actions right now, what could I do to respond in a way that would make Him/Her/Supreme Source/Creator proud of who I am as a reflection of Light, Love, Compassion, and Conscious Awareness?

5. **Express yourself!** Journal, create art, cry, laugh, and vocalize in ways such as chanting, singing, and screaming at the top of your lungs.

Physical exercise is another excellent option to move through your emotions in a healthy, natural way. Western medicine offers an ocean of prescription drugs to improve your mood. If you're currently using these, or considering this path, I encourage you to recognize the "quick fix" dilemma created by this path of "desensitizing" oneself. This cannot and will not provide you the long-term peace you deserve. There are natural herbal mood enhancers like kava kava, for instance, that you can utilize while you are still developing your physical strength, emotional balance, and mental clarity.

Sometimes you may find that you just need to step away. Leave without saying anything. This isn't necessarily polite, but if that is the best you can do, work with what you have. On the other hand, if you feel strong and in control of yourself, then you can formulate a response to the situation that is challenging you, one that will be win-win and generated from the compassion you have in your heart. Just know, either way, that you have attracted this situation into your life experience so you can grow and learn the lessons necessary to get to the next level.

Look for the message inside the mess!

Every moment is an opportunity to become more enlightened, more open and expanded. Continually choose that path and you will be free. According to Dr. Michael J. Lincoln, author of many books including *Messages in the Body*,

> Every condition in our lives exists because there is a need for it in one way or another, either on the time-space level or on the soul level or both. The symptoms, reactions or conditions are the outward effect of the inner condition of the individual.
>
> A specific sickness is the natural physical outcome of particular thought patterns and/or emotional disharmonies. They are coded messages from the body to the effect of what is happening and what needs to happen. In effect, then, illnesses and ailments teach

us, expand us, and move us on—if we can understand them and heed them.

There is a kind of "escalation chain" effect involved in this matter of consciousness distortions showing up in the body's malfunctioning. It starts out as psychological phenomena such as disturbing thoughts, wishes, fantasies, intentions, interpretations or repressions.

If these are ignored, avoided or resisted, it then moves to mild disruptions of our functioning such as fatigue, irritation reactions, or sleep pattern disruptions. If the situation continues to not be heeded, it then moves to acute physical disturbances like inflammations, wounds and minor accidents.

If we still don't get the message and we persist in the pattern of consciousness/functioning that is causing the problem, we move on to chronic conditions, where we receive a lasting reminder of our situation.

If we still stubbornly refuse to acknowledge our problem and to adjust our consciousness, the soul and/or the Cosmos will precipitate traumatic events such as accidents, assaults, lightning strikes and the like.

If all this fails, the situation deteriorates into irreversible physical changes or incurable processes. The individual then proceeds to descend into such outcomes as cancer or degenerative disorders like "Lou Gehrig's disease" or AIDS.

If the individual continues in their patterns even then, this development leads to death, the ultimate acknowledgement that we are not a separate "I" in a strictly physical world. We are conscious beings in a sea of consciousness, where the requirement is to be "at one with the One."

It should be noted that all illnesses and disorders are based on the same source: a deep sense of separation from God. The situation of being in a physical body in time-space lays the groundwork for this experience, and it then is exaggerated/exacerbated by non-optimal life experiences.*

In order to heal ourselves from physical pain and tension, we must feel our emotional pain simultaneously. If we work on only one of these aspects of who we are, instead of both, it will take much longer and be much more challenging.

Just like everything in life, we can take the easy road or the challenging path. After many years of taking the long route and swimming against the stream I learned this lesson the hard way.

Pranashama Yoga for Healing

Another goal of the Pranashama Yoga system is to help heal and bring wholeness to your life.

Healing (verb): to restore to purity or integrity; to make spiritually whole.

The story about the bicycle accident I was in and the ensuing ten-year process of healing it required is an illustration of what we attract to us that guides us to heal our life. I say "heal our life" because it is not just our physical body that is affected when we experience physical injury, illness, or disease.

Everything affects everything.

This is a fundamental principle to understand how we can be successful in the Journey to Joyful or the path to wholeness. It *starts by loving yourself.* It always starts there. If you love yourself, you will do whatever it takes to restore your health and happiness.

---

*Michael J. Lincoln, *Messages from the Body: Their Psychological Meaning* (Cool, California: Talking Hearts, 2006).

It has been a journey and a process to grow to love myself completely. And for many years, I was really ignorant about all the ways in which I wasn't loving myself. I would use positive habits to justify my negative habits that were hurting me. When I used to drink, I always told myself, "Well, I exercise and eat really healthy, so I deserve to let loose in at least this one area." And in some cases, this is okay, until it's not anymore. I recognize that for most of us, the path to loving ourselves is initially very slow. So, don't be too hard on yourself—you are where you are. And I assure you of one simple truth about your soul's development. You are exactly where you want to be!

The fundamental problem is: *by justifying our harmful negative habits, we live in delusion.* We are lying to ourselves. And worse yet, we waste the precious opportunity of living our truth. With a human body that typically lasts for less than one hundred years, we need to recognize how precious every moment is and proceed with this awareness to heal that which is out of balance in our lives and maximize the enjoyment of our time here. Not just for ourselves, for everyone we love.

Addictions are an outdated paradigm.

In a world resistant to change, we have to take matters into our own hands. Our culture fails to support our healing by literally encouraging us to sustain our addictions. I find it amazing that alcohol is not only legal throughout the majority of the world, it is actually encouraged as a cultural activity. This baffles me when I consider the immense amount of harm it creates in our lives with virtually no benefits. India is one of the rare countries I visited that has entire states that are "dry" non-alcohol states. India also has vast regions where people don't eat meat as well, so they live an entirely different lifestyle on many levels, but there's something that needs deeper exploration here. Let's examine our culture's three most common addictions.

Why are we eating, drinking, and smoking so much?

When I was a big drinker it came natural for me. Despite my petite frame, I had built up a tremendous tolerance and could drink most large men under the table. I was the champion of keg stands in high school! No joke. Sixty seconds in a handstand without coming up for a breath. (Now you can see where my yoga handstand and breathwork practice began!) All silliness aside, the point I am making is that while I was drinking a lot, my body was building up an immunity to the toxicity that I was ingesting, as best it could. After I quit, and I quit cold turkey for a full year, I couldn't tolerate much more than a few sips when I tried to go back. My system had become so clean and was moving toward wholeness so quickly (time is subjective here), that I haven't been able to drink much since. Now it's been almost seven years, a full life cycle has progressed for me, and I see the whole experience of drinking in a new light. Alcohol is a toxic poison to our body. *Webster's definition of intoxication: poisoning or the abnormal state induced by a chemical agent.* The same is true of the nicotine in cigarettes, and the sugar or MSG in junk food. Underneath the surface we discover the deeper reasons we drink, smoke, and overeat, in spite of our knowledge of the hazardous effects to our health.

The emotional reasons we drink, smoke, and overeat ...

Through my studies of yoga, chakras, *marmas*, meridians/energy points, and lines on the body, I have come to see the human design in an entirely new light. In addition to the chakras and *koshas* described, it is also important to discuss another Eastern approach to the human body. Traditional Chinese Medicine works with energy channels or meridians that run throughout the body. These channels correlate to our organ functions, and each channel has several points accessible through acupuncture and acupressure. Healing practitioners work with the various meridians to bring the body back into harmonious balance.

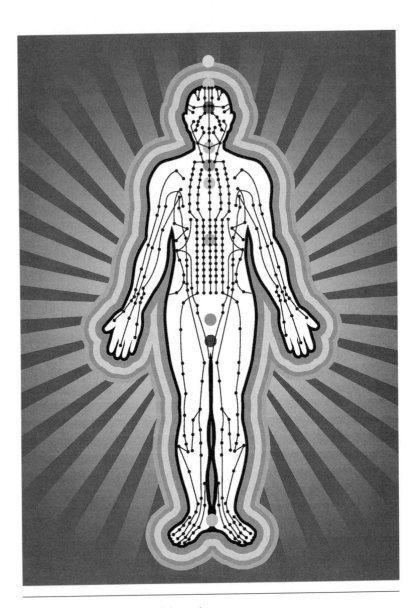

The Main Meridian Channels of the Body

According to Traditional Chinese Medicine, each organ has an emotion to which it corresponds. For example, the liver processes anger, the lungs process grief, and the stomach processes feelings of despair. See Appendix C for a complete list of organs and their corresponding emotions.

I bring these three organs into the picture to illustrate the root of what drives us to our addictions. We turn to alcohol, cigarettes, and excessive eating (among other addictions) to avoid feeling our emotions. I mentioned that alcohol was a constant for many years of my life. I used it to mask or avoid a deep-seated anger I felt toward men. I didn't know it at the time, and it wasn't until I stopped drinking that I realized I was carrying all this latent anger. Without my unconscious addiction (alcohol in this case) to turn to, I was forced to feel these feelings. A lot came up. I knew I had anger toward my father, but I was shocked to learn that I carried that into every relationship with every man I'd ever known. As I've healed this dynamic with my father and reconciled the emotional pattern I developed with him, I've opened myself to relating with greater freedom and love not only with men, but with everyone in my life.

A friend of mine quit smoking after more than ten years. He recently shared with me some powerful insights that support the idea that we turn to these toxic substances to avoid the toxic emotions that our addictions cover up. For his entire life he felt like he never received the love and affection he needed from his mother. He felt as though something was missing, that something was lost! Instead of feeling the heavy grief that resulted, he turned to smoking. He went on to replicate this dynamic with the feminine by dating women who were disinclined to being openly loving and affectionate. And even when they were, it was never enough. When he couldn't find what he needed in his partners (*which will never be the case; we must first connect with the self-love within!*), he turned to cigarettes and marijuana. As he entered more deeply into his yoga practice, he found his habitual addiction to nicotine and THC too toxic to continue doing both.

He came to a choice point. When he (wisely) cut smoking out of his life he discovered a well of grief just waiting to be processed. It warrants mention that he also discovered right around this time that he wasn't breast-fed as an infant. He recognized the oral fixation resultant from that early trauma, and the unconscious belief he developed that women could never provide him with what he needed. When he recognized the perpetual grief that this conditioned belief created, it became crystal clear to him that rather than turn back to the habit of smoking that comforted him in the past, his soul would best be served by embracing the beauty of the healing path to which this early trauma led him. To this day he credits his yoga practice to healing his relationship with his inner feminine, in addition to his now wonderfully harmonious relationship with his mother. And, of course, he is currently enjoying a new and deeply nourishing romantic relationship that transcends his old patterns.

A final example involves one of my clients who spent the majority of her life overweight and unhappy. She grew up in a very conservative household that offered little in the way of expressing love or offering support. This led her to feel inadequate and unworthy of love. She perpetuated this lie by covering her feeling of despair with excessive overeating. Whenever she looked in the mirror she would see what she falsely believed—someone inadequate by society's standards and therefore unworthy of love. She found yoga through my online videos and slowly began to discover her true Self, her body, and her feelings through regular *asana* practice. After a few months she went beyond doing yoga once a week and began to study on her own as well. Not only did she lose weight and feel more energized, she no longer feels the false sense of despair that plagued her for so many years.

These real-life examples illustrate why we make the unconscious choices that quickly turn into addictions. We turn to various substances that cover up the latent emotions we're afraid to feel. Where does this fear come from? Why are we conditioned to feel this way? The origins of our conditioned mind will be addressed in further detail in the next chapter about the mind, but we can appreciate with the above examples that the conditioned beliefs we carry about ourselves generate a life reality that mirrors these beliefs. Again and again the reflections of this universal truth shine through the countless testimonials of the transformation available in the practice of yoga.

> The more you depend on forces outside yourself, the more you are dominated by them.
>
> —*Harold Sherman*

Three Keys to Eliminating Addiction

... and successfully eliminating what is hurting you to awaken to a deeper appreciation for yourself and life in general

Meditation and the Observation of Thought. Fundamentally, this is where it all begins. When you quit something, whether it is drinking, smoking, overeating, laziness, or letting go of a codependent relationship, to name a few examples, you reprogram your subconscious mind to no longer need or want that thing, activity, or person in your life or at least not allow it to control your life. On a physical level, we crave what we are addicted to. We have emotional cords tied to these things, and spiritually, we are bonded as well. It is a process of cutting the cords on all levels and this begins in the mind. It is essential that you have a good journal to write down your thoughts as they arise for you. This will help when you feel drawn to relapse. Also, even if you do have a temporary relapse, keep coming back to your thoughts. Observe: is it a specific time of day, or is there a trigger that sends you into a relapse? You will learn about the Buddhist concept of *shenpa* in Chapter 3 of this book. That explains in detail the origin of triggered responses and offers suggestions for how to overcome them through meditation.

Find an accountability partner. When I quit drinking, it was easy, because I was really ready. Additionally, I was with a man who was in the same place in his life and we both did it together. We had had enough. It was clear that it was doing us more harm than good. We had both had run-ins with the law, jail time (only a few hours), and now we were committed to experiencing a higher vibration. We both wanted to create something real and impactful with our lives, and this bonded us in a powerful way. It was a process of eliminating the negative influences/friends and environments that were drawing us into the trap of habituation that led to the negative patterning we were ready to release. We had to reprogram our entire lifestyles, and it was easier to do this since we had each other. It is ideal if you are married, if your accountability partner is your spouse, or even your lover or best friend, since they are often the number-one influence upon your lifestyle choices. If this is not your situation, then ask those to whom you are close to please support you in your new lifestyle choices. I guarantee you will get overwhelming responses of positivity and encouragement.

Replace the Habits. This is key. If you typically find yourself drinking at a bar on a Friday night, or even having drinks at home, or whatever your issue is that you're ready to let go of, you must find another activity that is equally enjoyable for you to replace the other. I recommend exercise, yoga, meditation, singing, dancing, and connecting with nature in various ways like camping, hiking, walking on the beach— anything that gets your body moving and away from what's sucking you into the trap. If your old friends are not interested or ready to let go of these negative habits, just find other ways in which you can connect with them. This happened to me. When I decided to quit drinking, it led to a complete transition in friends. This was hard at first. There was a period of time when my only friends were my sisters and my boyfriend. That was fine, however, since I was so excited about the new level of energy, enthusiasm, and excitement about life and my future that I was ready to move on and up from the old habits, thus I was grateful to let them go. *Embrace releasing of the old to welcome in the new.* It will serve you richly for the entirety of your life.

The fastest way to freedom is to feel your feelings.

—Gita Bellin

The Three Emotional Prison Keepers

#1. Expectations: the act or action of looking forward; mental attitude of one who anticipates.

Placing expectations upon people, objects, or events will inevitably lead to suffering. Suffering is the opposing frequency to happiness, joy, and bliss—life's greatest gifts and the aspiration of the Pranashama Yoga path. Remember, you are always at choice in how you perceive the events of your life.

There is no way to control the result or "effect" of that which is outside yourself. When we place our intention upon something in an expectant way, and it doesn't deliver the goods, we are usually "let down," disappointed, and hurt. These emotions lead us away from happiness and further from our goals in life. The more time we spend in these painful and negative emotional states, the less we are living in alignment with our highest truth, which is otherwise joyful and free.

Additionally, when we spend time wallowing in these negative emotions, we block the flow of positive experiences from entering our lives. This is perhaps the greatest reason to practice living without expectation. It benefits everyone involved.

Here's an example: Let's say you have an expectation that for your birthday your partner or friends will honor your special day with a party and many gifts. The day arrives and it appears that no one even remembers that this is your special day! From morning until night, you do not receive even one phone call. Your partner appears to go about the daily routine as if it is just any other day. You naturally feel let down, hurt, or unloved. In that state of emotion, nothing feels good. As the evening approaches, your partner doesn't even mention a birthday dinner and you grow more and more upset, hurt, and angry. These feelings rob you of your day and the joy of living.

On the contrary, if you were to carry on with gratitude, celebrating in your own way without a single expectation, the day will be blissful and joyous, regardless of whether or not anyone else acknowledges the blessing of your birth. Residing in a state of gratitude and contentment with simplicity, nourishing your heart and soul for yourself, and in recognition that you are one with the Supreme Source—that alone is a continuous celebration. Then every day becomes your birthday!

Returning to the example of the birthday and the approaching evening, all day long you've been waiting, in anticipation, for someone/something to fulfill you—hoping, wishing, *expecting* someone to honor you. Externalizing your energy in all of this, you move further and further away from the Source, *which is within you* and has the ability to fulfill you beyond your wildest imagination. So, you spend your birthday, for the most part, in a less than blissful emotional state of separation. Now evening has come. Your partner brings home a generic birthday card, a small cake for the family, and a small bouquet of flowers he picked up from the local supermarket on his way home. . . . Now what? Does your mood improve because you've moved from receiving nothing into a space of receiving something? Or, do you remain disconnected from your Bliss Channel because *what* you receive doesn't live up to your *expectation?* Now, it may be obvious there wasn't as much thought and consideration put into your birthday as you might prefer or feel you deserve, but this is all a setup! When we attach our happiness to the behavior of others, we will inevitably be let down. However, when you perceive life without expectation and live in a state of non-attachment, everything is perfect, everything is divine. As we play out our roles in this divine theatre, we must remain open to what IS, staying present with our innate gratitude and unconditional love.

> If you would learn the secret of right relations look only for
> the divine in people and things, and leave all the rest to God.
>
> —J. Allen Boone

#2. Attachment: the state of being attached; the feeling that binds a person.

We naturally become attached to people and things from day one. As infants, we are dependant on our mother's love and nourishment. Without it we would perish. Therefore, we develop limbic attachments from our very inception. Albeit necessary in order to bond people together, attachments will eventually lead us to emotional states that perpetuate our suffering. Life is full of one paradox after another, and this one proves enormously fruitful when we transcend the subjective experience by feeling our feelings completely, and objectively observing them without attachment. On our Journey to Joyful, we will consistently attract situations that show us where we are attached. These are prime opportunities to let go in surrender to that which is greater than our egoistic needs and desires.

> Men are disturbed not by things that happen but by their
> opinion of the things that happen.
>
> —Epictetus

How do we know if we are attached to something? Try this. Think of something in your life that you absolutely can't imagine living without. Close your eyes—really SEE it in your mind. Now write it down. It can be a person, a material possession, or even something that isn't yours, but that you long to have (such as a dream, goal, or wish).

When we identify what we are attached to (generally, the list is long for most of us), we're able to see what is holding us captive. I believe it is totally acceptable to have love for things, people, and the ideas and dreams we envision. On the other hand, however, it is not nourishing to our soul when our attachment to these things prevents us from fully accepting the present moment. This is where attachments become detrimental. We have to remember that life isn't about the destination, it's about the journey. *As with all things in the physical plane, nothing is permanent, and the only thing we can truly count on is change.* Things come and go, people are born and die and move in and out of our lives. The dreams and goals of today will either materialize or evolve into something different with time. If we become rigidly attached to any of this, we set ourselves up for the inevitable suffering that will ensue when the thing, person, or idea flows out of our lives, or our desire for it shifts.

Here's an example. Most people spend a tremendous amount of energy seeking a partner with whom to share their life. Attachment begins at the very origin of thought. A vision of what this person will look like, how they will behave, and even what they will enjoy doing begins to formulate in the mind, and that establishes the criteria from which the "search" is then based. It can be powerful to visualize our potential life partner to attract him or her into our lives, but when we become attached to the exact "how" and "what," we are opening ourselves to being let down. Then if someone comes along who doesn't fit our mental mold, we may automatically reject him or her because we are attached to this partner "looking" a certain way. This person, who doesn't fit our specific mental idea for an ideal mate, may turn out to possess traits beyond our constructed vision of ideal.

Conversely, if a person who "fits" our mental mold comes along, but he or she doesn't show the same level of mutual interest in us, we may fall prey to the suffering that comes from being attached to "having found the perfect mate" and the pain of being rejected. The letdown can be heart-breaking, thus perpetuating the cycle of suffering until you are finally freed from the prison that attachment can create. It is key to remember that we can maintain a genuine enthusiasm and love for what is, in the present moment, enjoying it with gratitude for all the blessings in our lives. Whether you're at the peak or the valley of any given wave, remember that this too shall pass. Trust always, whatever it is, that it is always for our highest good. When we return continually to the present moment and our centered awareness within it, we remember that we are eternally connected to the Supreme Source that lives within us.

> As long as you are unable to access the power of the Now,
> every emotional pain that you experience leaves behind a
> residue of pain that lives on in you.

> —Eckhart Tolle

A personal example: When I was twenty-four, I met a beautiful man named Joseph, with whom I fell in love. He was a runway model in Miami, and a lifelong student of Nin Jutsu. We had so much fun together. We grappled and he taught me the way of the Ninja Masters. I taught him yoga, and we shared a love for dancing that was so sweet and innocent. He was a powerful reflection for me, mirroring many years of unhealed childhood sadness and fragmented inner-child issues that wouldn't allow him to surrender to love completely.

True to my character at the time, I fell into a state of attachment that led to the inevitable suffering that follows. He was so wrapped up in his personal life and the drama of his own story, he would go weeks without returning my calls. This behavior thus allowed me to fall into my own story. I was operating under the personal lie at the time that "men can never give me what I want and/or need. And that nothing men can do is ever enough."

Being the avid communicator that I am, it was agonizing for me. I would feel crushed when he didn't call, taking it personally, as if he didn't like me; or I would project assumptions that he must be interested in other women. Since beautiful women surrounded him during his modeling shoots, it was a reasonable assumption, but very disturbing nonetheless. We'd go weeks without seeing each other and days without any communication.

Just like many people, I was *attached* to my own ideas about what a relationship should look, feel, and taste like, and this one was not matching those expectations. Here I was operating under two of the emotional prison keepers and not clear about how to break free. I found solace in my yoga practice and attending workshops with Master Teachers from around the world. In these trainings I learned so much more than how to perfect yoga poses. I learned how to finally love myself completely and feel whole.

Know that Love is the most powerful energy in the Universe.

—Sanaya Roman, Soul Love

#3. Judgment: the mental or intellectual process of forming an opinion or evaluation by discerning or comparing.

The mind loves to judge and compare and stir up all kinds of negative emotions such as envy, greed, scarcity, jealously, etc. As we walk through life we judge everything including ourselves, others, things, ideas, the past, present, and future. We compare ourselves to others and to illusionary images of a socially created concept of perfection. This is another source of great suffering in our lives if our minds are always being plagued with thoughts of inferiority, lack, and what is not present for us now. We live in a state that is seldom nourishing for our heart and soul. This mental state triggers negative emotions that lead to a compulsive repetition of endless suffering.

First of all, it is essential to know that you are perfect as you are. My conviction that this was not so was another personal lie I had to release years ago.

Like many people, I was always comparing myself to my friends and squandering my energy under the harsh scrutiny of my own judgment that I was "less than." I took the approach of pushing myself to be better than I could even imagine possible. How? I used my limiting beliefs to empower me to become stronger, better, and more successful than those I was comparing myself with—not to compete with them, but actually to prove my own critical judgment wrong. After years of that, I found myself still falling into a state of suffering in certain circumstances. For instance, in the presence of a beautiful friend I'd question how I looked. Or upon learning of others who had been blessed with the reward of success, I wondered if my own efforts were good enough.

These judgments and instances of self-criticism would trigger negative emotional spiraling that I could not escape. It would come as the sensation of a constriction in my heart center, almost as if I were being squeezed in the chest, making it difficult to breathe. I'd know immediately the effect this was having on me, since it was such a physical experience. And in a serious effort to raise my emotional experience into one of openness and free-flowing love, I came to understand that it was this judgment and comparison that was causing the pain in my chest. If left un-reconciled, this would lead to tension in the shoulders, upper back, and neck. After a period of time, if it is still not dealt with, such an emotion and its accompanying physical effects can evolve into something more serious, for example, injury in this area of your body, heart or lung problems, and disease.

Continuing with this specific example, I notice that people tend to reach for a smoke to ease this tension in their heart. The smoke can be either tobacco or marijuana, or some other drug or food that may numb the discomfort, if only for a short time. Referring back to our basic understanding of the energetic anatomy, meridians, and chakras of the body, we can once again appreciate the correlation between where you are experiencing physical discomfort and the major energetic points that are being blocked. When you can start to see yourself in this way, you will be able to recognize which habits you have created in order to avoid feeling these emotions fully and to liberate yourself from their unconscious effects.

Here's an exercise to test if something is affecting you in a negative way: Stop what you are doing and close your eyes. Think about something that you *do* or some way that you *are*, in comparison to someone whom you feel embodies the mastery that you desire. How does it make you feel to see them as better than you in that way? Do you feel any constriction in your heart center at the thought of this? What thoughts arise with this exercise? Try writing them down.

The key here is, when you do become aware of yourself at this level of depth, you must then have the proper tools to make the shift into a more holistic pattern. In the example above, when I find myself judging or comparing myself to others, I try to stop, take a few breaths, and remind myself of my own accomplishments or other positive attributes that I embody.

Our deepest fear is that we are powerful beyond measure.
It is our light, not our darkness that most frightens us.
We ask ourselves,
Who am I to be brilliant, gorgeous, talented, fabulous?
Actually, who are you *not* to be?
You are a child of God.
Your playing small does not serve the world.
There is nothing enlightened about shrinking so that other people won't feel insecure around you.
We are all meant to shine, as children do.
We were born to make manifest the glory of God that is within us.
It's not just in some of us; it's in everyone.
And as we let our own light shine, we unconsciously give other people permission to do the same.
As we are liberated from our own fear, our presence automatically liberates others.

—*Marianne Williamson*, A Return to Love

The most common tool for overriding doubts and fears is positive affirmations. Recognize the polarity frequency, the opposite emotion or quality, to whatever negativity you're feeling, and simply choose it. An additional approach to improve your self-worth and self-esteem is to remind your subconscious of all the best qualities that you possess with confidence, as often as you can. This technique of realigning thought patterns and quieting the voice of negativity is an effective strategy to strengthen personal power.

Loving Myself

In my life, I was always searching externally for someone to complete me—to fulfill my longing for love. In some romantic delusion, I had always wanted a partner but never questioned why. When I recognized within myself that I was seeking to fulfill something that I felt was missing, it created a profound shift in my path. Through the study and practice of yoga I have learned that we all possess both masculine and feminine within ourselves. We have the tendency, by virtue of our gender, to operate predominantly from one more than the other. This is most often perceived as "normal" since that is how the majority of people operate. Additionally, by virtue of our upbringing we have the tendency to become strong in some areas of our character and weaker in others. Thus, it is not surprising that we find ourselves seeking a partner to "fulfill us" or "be our other half" by embodying that which we lack or wish we possessed within ourselves.

We attract mirrors of ourselves.

We tend to attract people to mirror what we are currently lacking within. Throughout the path of life, ideally, we are continually moving toward wholeness, completeness, and union with the Supreme Source. Because of this, we will attract potential partners who reflect back to us what we need to heal, balance, and strengthen in ourselves—until we become whole. At that point, we can attract our twin flame or soul mate and enjoy a peaceful co-creative partnership that benefits all humankind.

What is the solution?

When we live in a state of presence, openness, appreciation, and love for WHAT IS, we transcend the suffering that results from the attachment to fulfilling our desires. Letting go of projections into the future about what *may* come and releasing the memories from the past about what *once was* or *was not*, we are FREE.

How do we cultivate this state of Presence?

Technique: The most powerful techniques to help cultivate presence and relinquish my attachments I have learned through the practice of yoga, breathwork, and meditation or the conscious observation of thought. When we stop to breathe, slowly and with awareness, we force ourselves to be still. In Pranashama Yoga I teach people to focus on their breath. Close your eyes. Listen to the sound it makes as you inhale, filling your lungs and expanding your heart center. Notice the pause between the inhale and the exhale, and find peace in that stillness. As you exhale, allow stress, tension, or negative emotions to flow out of you, as if you are washing yourself with your breath. Again, notice the space you create between the exhale and the next inhale. Witness if your mind wanders away from the breath and begins entertaining thoughts. Just watch, observing where these thoughts take you. Ask yourself the following questions:

Are these thoughts triggering a negative state of emotions based upon fears, projections, or judgments?

If the answer is yes, relax into the breath even more deeply and consciously let these emotions go. Don't be surprised if they don't exit easily. In the beginning of your practice thoughts tend to have more power until you tame the mind and gain control over your thoughts. *Recognizing that they are powerless until you give them power frees you from their potential to trigger the negative emotional sensations.* Then you can relax into knowing that your true self lives beyond the limited realm of thoughts and emotions—your soul is limitless, luminous, and completely free. At your essence, you are Divine in nature and One with the Supreme Source.

Pranayama Breathing Exercises

This is a perfect time to introduce the fundamental and essential practice of *pranayama*. This is the fourth limb in the Ashtanga eight-limb system created by C.E. Patanjali.

Breath is your link to life, the direct connection to your spirit. It is upon this awareness that the entire system of Pranashama Yoga is based. Calming the mind and connecting with breath, we can move beyond the dual nature of our lives into a unified field, a non-dual current of unconditional love and joy. This is the gateway to accessing the Bliss Channel. Additionally, conscious awareness and the ability to control the breath will increase your energy levels naturally, improve your sleeping patterns, and detoxify your lungs (along with many other benefits).

Pranayama is a Sanskrit word meaning literally "restraint of the *prana* or breath." The word is composed of two parts: *prana*, life force or vital energy, particularly, the breath; and *ayama*, to suspend or restrain. It is often translated as "control of the life force." The breath is regulated and controlled through the practice of breathing exercises. The duration of inhalation, retention, and exhalation of breath is regulated with the aim of strengthening and cleansing the nervous system and increasing a person's source of life energy. *Pranayama* practice also makes the mind calmer and more focused.

Pranayama is a vitally essential inclusion into the Pranashama Yoga system. A few of the most commonly shared techniques include:

1. **Nadi Shodhana,** alternate nostril breathing. This balances both brain hemispheres and brings the mind and body into harmony and balance. It's perfect for people who experience anxiety or stress or feel imbalanced in any way. The core objective is to clean up (*shodhan*) all energy lines (*nadis*) inside our bodies so that there is no blockage left and the life energy can freely flow throughout all levels to deliver the best health condition to the practitioner.

2. **Kapalabhati,** fire breathing, is a very active, forced exhalation with a passive inhalation. To exhale, the belly quickly pumps into the spine, forcing the air out of the nose (like trying to blow out a candle through your nose). Place a hand on your belly to feel it actively pumping. Play with the tempo (45–60 exhalations/30 seconds), but keep a steady rhythm. Start with 2–3 rounds of 30 exhalations, and gradually increase the number of exhalations if comfortable.

3. **Kumbhaka Breath,** breath retention; lung expansion breath; pronounced *kuhm-BAH-kah*. *Kumbha* = pot (a traditional image of the human torso as a container for the breath with two "openings" at the throat and base of the pelvis). The practice of this technique will improve the quality of your life on many levels. The ability to hold more air in your lungs for a longer duration of time will raise your pranic levels considerably.

4. **Ujjai Breath,** or victorious breath. This is the breath we practice while flowing in Pranashama Vinyasa practice. Best known for the deep hissing sound that is created by slightly blocking the back of the throat, this type of breath utilizes deep inhales through the nose into the upper chest and lungs while engaging the lower belly and maintaining a strong core with *bandhas* (energy locks) engaged.

5. **Belly Breathing.** This is the simplest one to practice. It is exactly how it sounds. You simply breathe deeply in through your nose into your belly. Each inhale expands your belly like a balloon. Each exhale releases the air and allows the balloon to deflate, drawing your navel toward your spine. This technique induces deep relaxation and peace while releasing stress. It's wonderful to practice *mantras* while lying on your back (e.g. inhale "love," exhale "anger").

This list is by no means conclusive. There are many other beneficial *pranayama* breathing exercises available, all of which facilitate movement through the emotional traumas we hold in our body and the mental blockages they create. Of these disturbing emotions, judgment is arguably the most rampant—not just of others, but also of ourselves. Objectively speaking, there's really no difference.

Strengthening Your Chakras

Affirmations to Strengthen Your Solar Plexus Chakra/Personal Power

I am Divine.

I am a Strong Powerful Woman (or Man).

I am here for a purpose.

I embody Strength, Openness, and Happiness.

We are all One; I am above no one and below no one.

The attributes I possess are unique and powerful.

My soul is strong and desires to evolve.

I feel powerful, ready to face whatever life has to offer.

I recognize that all I attract is of my doing, to help me evolve to my highest potential.

Chakra Empowering Practices

Other techniques that are equally and powerfully effective include exercise and the strengthening of your core. If you understand the energy centers or chakras that comprise your body, you can begin to see where you may be weak and blocked or strong and balanced. You can take the Chakra Personality Survey on page 123 in the appendix of this book to get a snapshot into the current condition of your energy centers. My personal example, about the judgment and comparison I used to experience, is a textbook third- and fourth-chakra imbalance.

Comparison and feeling "less than" is linked to a weak or blocked third chakra. This energy center aligns with your confidence and personal power and is called the *Manipura*, located at the solar plexus between your heart and your navel. This is the core of your body. In Pranashama Yoga, we use yoga *asanas* and sequences to specifically strengthen, tone, and unblock the *Manipura*, as well as all other chakras in the body.

The other chakra in need of opening in this example is the fourth chakra, heart center (*Anahata*). When this chakra is blocked or out of balance, our feelings are very sensitive and we take things too seriously. We lose compassion for ourselves and for others. This often generates a feeling of heartache or constriction in the heart center. The best practices to open and balance this area are breathing exercises (*pranayama*) into the heart center.

Pause for a moment and take some long, slow, deep breaths directly into your chest. Feel yourself unhook from any sensations not connected to unconditional love. You are at choice with how you relate to all energy that arises. Choose love and be free of the outdated patterns. Among yoga *asanas* we use back bending, neck stretching, and shoulder stretches to help open and balance the fourth chakra. Chanting, singing, and other sound vibrations also help. And perhaps most effective of all is to give love.

All too often we give in order to get, i.e., we place conditions on the recipients of whatever we're giving. I did this for you, so you owe me. Let's be honest, we've all done this. This will unavoidably take us back into the expectation/disappointment dilemma we've already discussed. *When we give love freely, generously, and without expecting anything in return, this compassionate act opens the heart chakra like nothing else.* I like to call it "Relaxing into Openness." Trust me, it works! And besides, it's good karma to give when someone is in need. Even if that person never repays you, the universe will take care of you tenfold!

Healing the Inner Child

Inner Child is a concept used in popular psychology and analytical psychology to denote the childlike aspect of a person's psyche, especially when viewed as an independent entity. Frequently, the term is used to address subjective childhood experiences and the lingering effects of one's childhood. "Inner child" also refers to all the emotional memories and experiences stored in the brain from our earliest years. The Twelve-step Program recovery movement considers healing the inner child to be one of the essential stages in recovery from addiction, abuse, trauma, or post-traumatic stress disorder. In the 1970s, the inner-child concept emerged alongside the clinical concept of codependency (initially called Adult Children of Alcoholics Syndrome).

In order to access the ultimate human experience, we must eventually acknowledge where we have been wounded throughout our lives, from childhood, adolescence, and adulthood, as well as from past-life karma carried into this lifetime.

Many people try to block out memories from their past that were painful, in an attempt to "move on" with their lives. This act of denial and repressed pain in the heart and consciousness is an underestimated cause of much of our suffering. Even when the memory is not present on the conscious level, we find ourselves acting from habitual patterns that tend to attract situations that continually trigger these negative and painful emotions.

Entire books have been written about the topic of healing the inner child, but I will explain briefly the essential nature of this inner work. Left unhealed, the wounded inner child will affect your life dramatically in every way.

Not everyone has the opportunity to grow up in a perfect nurturing family. And even those people who were lucky enough to be born to parents who were loving and supportive find that it is impossible to live in this world of duality free from inner-child trauma or wounds. When we address this aspect of our psyche, we can create major improvements in the quality of our life experience. Healing the inner child is like lifting a huge weight off your shoulders, out of your heart, and away from your daily life.

As we mature and grow older, we often disregard all that our body has accumulated over the years. Each and every experience has left an imprint on our mind, heart, and soul, and all that remains unprocessed gets *stored* in the body. This includes the wounds and traumas, both physical and emotional, from our infancy until the present. When conflict arises in a relationship, this is a perfect reminder. Our close friends, colleagues, and loved ones trigger in us what remains unhealed on a psychological level. We are seldom aware of the origin of the emotional reactions we have when conflict arises, or even the inner conflict we experience. Instead of taking responsibility for our feelings, we look to blame others. This is the first sign that we are either unaware or in denial of our inner-child issues.

How do we heal the inner child?

Every time I recognized myself falling into an unconscious pattern that was not supporting my highest vision for my life, I knew I was defaulting to and acting from my hurt inner child. In my experience, I have used several methods to heal my inner-child issues.

As long as we are in a human body, we are forming emotional cords with the people we come into contact with. Beyond just the physical, we bond throughout the five levels of the *koshas*. The more time we spend with someone, the stronger the bonds/cords grow to be. This is part of the reason why our love and appreciation increase for those with whom we spend a great deal of time or even much of our life. For all intents and purposes, we become addicted to their presence, their subtle vibration in our lives. This is also the reason it is so hard to let them go if the course of our life path requires us to do so. This is attachment in action and a perfect illustration of the importance of practicing non-attachment.

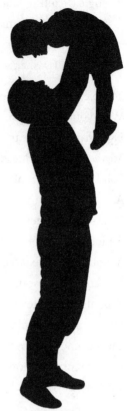

Inner-child healing work takes place within your mind, heart, and soul. It is advisable to have a trained professional to guide you through the inner-child healing meditations and practices. Following is a short list of therapies, as well as contact information for practitioners I highly recommend.

- Emotional Cord Cutting
- Rebirthing/Conscious Breathing (Sula DePaula: www.sulade-paula.com)
- Loving Relationships Training (Sula DePaula)
- Inner Child/Heart-Guided Meditations (Sanaya Roman: www.orindaben.com)

- Yogic Chanting Practices (Wah!: www.wahmusic.com, Snatam Kaur: www.snatamkaur.com)
- Forgiveness Therapy (Sula DePaula)
- Self Love (Dashama Konah Gordon: www.Dashama.com)

You blend your heart center's jewel
With your soul's jewel.
Light from your heart center
Moves up to your head center.
You know the serenity
And oneness of love.
Your soul activates
A hidden point of light
In your solar plexus center.
You know your soul's will to love.
You raise solar plexus energy
into your heart center
and surrender to love.
Light circulates among your heart centers.
You love as your soul.

—*Sanaya Roman*, Soul Love

Short Inner-Child Guided Meditation Practice

First, allow your body to relax. You can either be seated or lying down. I recommend the latter. Get comfortable and draw your awareness to your breath. With every inhale, think to yourself "I am," then as you exhale think "relaxed" and allow any tension to melt out of your mind and body as you exhale out all your cares. Take 10–20 deep slow breaths into your belly and repeat the above *mantra*. Allow your heart and mind to relax so you may merge with your soul during this meditation, uninterrupted by the thoughts and emotions from the day.

When you feel very relaxed, visualize yourself standing in a field somewhere. The sun is shining and in the distance you see a child, any age you might visualize between infancy and adolescence. The child is walking toward you. Notice anything about this child that may seem unusual. Perhaps this child is walking with a limp or hunched forward, perhaps running toward or away from you. Just observe and allow the child to continue to come closer until you are facing each other.

Now notice if there is anything about this inner child that is unusual or noteworthy. Perhaps the child is crying or laughing, smiling or frowning. How do the child's eyes look? Does the child appear to be happy or troubled? Allow for any and all emotions to arise without restraint. Bond with this child. Reach out and hold the child's hand. Lead the child (which is you!) walking, running, dancing, or flying up a small mountain.

When you get to the top, visualize the valley down below. To the left is your past, where you have been and what you have been through. Send healing love and forgiveness to all that exists in the past for you and this child. Allow the feeling of love to radiate from within you.

Now looking forward, you see the valley directly below, which represents the present time. Send forgiveness and healing love out to anything or anyone whom you feel needs it in your present life scenario. Now, turn to the child and give the child a warm heart-to-heart embrace. Feel the connection between yourself and the aspect of you that is present here in this child and all that he or she represents in your life right now.

Finally, with your inner child's hand in yours, turn to the right and see the vast valley that stretches out beyond your vision. This is the future you have in front of you. Open all your senses. See the beauty of the slanting rays of sunshine illuminate the valley below. Hear the soft vibration of the birds chirping. Feel the warm breeze blowing. Taste and smell the precious sweetness of this moment. Hold it in your heart. Release any pain or sadness about the past. Allow the child to forgive and be forgiven. And in turn, you may forgive and be forgiven for all things and in all ways. Now inhale deeply and feel the love that radiates from within your heart toward this child. Take as much time as you can to be present with all that arises. Feel your emotions. Know that the truth in you is whole and complete.

> Be like a very small joyous child, living gloriously in the ever present NOW, without a single worry or concern about even the next moment in time.
>
> —Eileen Caddy, cofounder of Findhorn

A Personal Example of Inner-Child Issues

Just after my high school graduation, I found myself living with my father for the first time since I was twelve years old. It was the biggest growth opportunity of my life. Here I am, living in a small apartment with a man I hardly know, and what I do know I genuinely don't like and completely distrust. He became a mirror for all the pain and suffering I felt in my heart, and the source of the subconscious anger I felt toward men. The strange part of the story is, I never even realized I had this in me until he brought it out—like a tidal wave!

We fought. A lot. I found myself reverting back to the words my mother would use when yelling at him when we were kids. Every fiber of my being wanted to move out and not live with him. As fate (and my higher Self!) would have it, I had no other option at the time.

So I stayed. And I cooked in the proverbial fire. An interesting thing happens when you come face to face with the darkest shadow aspect of yourself: when you allow it to arise, and you embrace it fully, it can heal.

After a period of time my anger started to subside. I slowly addressed each aspect of my inner child that held anger, resentment, jealousy, or hurt feelings toward my experiences with my father, mother, sisters, friends, and most importantly, with myself. I breathed through it all. I cried, I screamed, I sobbed, I laughed at myself, I forgave myself. I forgave all of them.

I wrapped it all in forgiveness and I let it all go.

It was an extraordinary process of exploration. And honestly, looking back, I loved every moment of it. I wouldn't trade that experience for anything. It made me a much more loving person. All of my relationships improved as a result of that inner-child healing work, and for that I am eternally grateful.

> The most difficult thing but an essential one is to love Life, to love even while one suffers, because Life is All. Life is God—and to love Life means to love God.
>
> —Leo Tolstoy

Embrace Your Shadow

Through the practice of yoga, we are learning to embrace all sides of ourselves—the dark and the light, and all emotions as well. We just keep letting go of our self-imposed limitations until we are completely free. And in that space of freedom, we can be clear about what we want, what we are here to do, and how we can best be of service to humanity while we are alive. Every time we practice meditation or step onto the yoga mat, we have the opportunity to observe our thoughts and emotions that arise. Through time, we are able to see things for what they are and not act, and to react or respond—or not—from a hurting inner-child experience. In the meantime, when we do notice ourselves reacting from that place, all we have to do is stop, breathe, and let it go.

Awakening the Heart Centers

There are several ways in which you can awaken the Heart Centers to ultimately have access to a higher and deeper sensation of Love in your life. It is important that we utilize all avenues, and not depend upon others to be our source of love. Ultimately we must discover and access the deep well of expansive openness that allows us to feel love from within. It is the only way we can come together with others on the Earth plane and effectively feel love with no expectations, judgment, or attachment.

> There's no transformation of the Earth without your
> transformation.
> —J. Krishnamurti

The Connection Between the Three Heart Centers

According to Sanaya Roman, from her profoundly healing book Soul Love, there are three heart centers. The primary Heart Center/Heart Jewel is located at the heart chakra, in the center of your chest. The other two heart centers are located above and below the heart chakra, at the crown of the head and the solar plexus. It is through these centers that we are able to draw upon our inner solar light (the light of the soul), get in touch with our inner child, and access the power and love of the Supreme Source as well as angels, light beings, and spirit guides. It is through working with these subtle realms that we explore an even wider field to heal our deep inner wounds and become free from the constricted feelings they have placed on our lives and in our hearts.

Thousands of years ago, it was a little different.

Since I have been an avid student and teacher of yoga for many years, I feel it is important for readers new to yoga or any type of heart awakening that I include a little background information about the yogic methods specifically, and then dive into the various other ways in which one may awaken the heart centers.

In the earliest years of exploration of human consciousness, yogis attained enlightenment by sitting and meditating and chanting in caves alone for years. This is effective for accessing the deepest and broadest experiences of love, since it is through mental clarity and stillness that we truly access the sea of love from within. However, these days it is less practical to do it that way. Most people in modern society choose to be householders and raise a family. We are actually born and raised to have a whole plethora of responsibilities that make it all but impossible to even consider a life of renunciation. Centuries ago, the yogis didn't have television, the Internet, cell phones, let alone a capitalist economy to deal with! For this reason, we have to modernize our approach to these ancient practices and allocate time differently in our dedication to awakening our heart centers. This limited-time concept is often the number-one excuse for not delving into this practice of healing your life. The initial reactions can be: *"I don't have the time for that."* *"I'm FINE."* Or *"I have no problems."*

These are all common responses that people come up with when approached about the potential of getting clear, healing their life, or what I like to refer to as "becoming clear light." It is the ego and pride that keep us from accessing the Bliss Channel and attaining the highest level of happiness. For some reason we like to fool ourselves into believing that everyone else is crazy and we are victims in an unfair world. This type of perspective is nothing other than self-created delusion that perpetuates our suffering (anger, frustration, loneliness, separation, etc.). Until we wake up and realize the truth—that every difficult situation is our meditation—we will resist the very concept, let alone the experience of unlimited bliss and expanded openness available to us at all times. We have to do the work as it arises, and the work is internal. When we resist diving into and connecting with our inner self, we resist growth, we resist healing, and we resist accessing our innate feelings of love and joy. What are we afraid of feeling? Why are we so resistant to feeling the enormity of our self-love?

There is no fear in love; for perfect love casteth out fear.

—I John 4:18

Three Levels of Love

There are three levels of Love in the human life experience.

1. First we must learn to love ourselves.

This is often the most difficult task because we spend our entire lifetime accumulating negative beliefs about ourselves! Our parents, siblings, friends, community, schoolmates, co-workers, and the culture at large have shaped who we are in such a way that we don't realize how far from our authentic self we truly are.

When we look in the mirror, we don't even see the same person that other people see when they look at us. All we see is our flaws or the ways in which we would like to be different. We constantly compare ourselves to others, basically ensuring that we will never measure up to some ideal of perfection that doesn't even exist. We operate under the assumption that everyone is judging us, and this creates a great deal of self-consciousness, as well as insecurity. These are all third chakra/solar plexus imbalances and weaknesses that are directly connected to the heart chakra's ability to grow stronger, larger, and more radiantly alive with Love.

Ten Ways to Access the Expansive Openness of Love from Within

Inner-Child healing/meditations

Devotionally chanting/singing spiritual music, from the heart

Pranayama: yogic breathing techniques to connect spiritual and physical human life experience, among other purposes

Crystal healing therapy, listening to resonant sound or healing music

Eating living foods and consuming only what will support and nourish you energetically

Spending time in direct communion with nature and her infinite intelligence

Yoga *Asanas* (back-bending and shoulder openers especially, while breathing into your heart centers)

Conscious connected breath therapy and loving relationship training

Karma Yoga: selfless service

Going on a retreat or vacation getaway

2. Next we learn how to truly love others.

Relationships can be both the most rewarding and the most challenging aspect of human existence. Our relationships are often the training ground that prepares us for the path to awakening our heart centers. We tend to attract mirrors into our lives that reflect back to us both our strengths and weaknesses, in order to help us grow to the next level of our potential.

When we practice patience, compassion, and empathy we are able to be more loving to others. We put ourselves in their shoes and see from their eyes. Everyone is working on something, so it is important to keep this in mind when we are interacting with others as well as in our more complex relationships. To experience harmony and peace within our lives, we must master the art of loving relationships.

Love is patient, love is kind,
Love does not insist on its own way.
Love bears all things, believes all things,
Hopes all things, endures all things.
Love never fails.

—I *Corinthians* 13:4–8

Learn to read the emotion (energy in motion) of others.

This may be one of the simplest things to say, and yet not so simple to act upon. The truth is, we cannot read the energy of others until we become sensitive to our own energy.

How do we become more sensitive to our own energy? Through the practice of yoga and meditation, we begin to become more connected with our senses. The yogic term is *pratyahara* (retraction of the senses). This is the fifth limb in the eight-limb system called Ashtanga Yoga.

Pratyahara refers to the ability to operate from a state of witness consciousness, observing the actions and energetic happenings around us (and within us!) without becoming caught up in them. We are aware without being affected. From this state of *pratyahara*, we are able to respond with calm presence and objectivity in all situations. This may be one of the most important practices of yoga, as it allows us to be in the world and not *of* the world. We can know what is happening all around us and discern between what is beneficial to get involved with, and what will be a waste of time and energy.

Over time, as you practice yoga and meditation, you will become energetically sensitive. You accomplish this with practice and by "getting clear" with yourself, which will in turn enable you to be clear about what others are feeling as well. This is invaluable in life, since it will enable you to move toward people who are radiating a warm, loving vibration and to walk away from those who are either energy vampires or just radiating cold, negative vibrations.

When you master this art, you will find yourself surrounded by love and light all the time. You simply won't be interested in being around people who don't match your frequency. You may eventually notice your circle of friends changing for the better!

Humanity is under great pressure to evolve because it is our only chance of survival as a race. This will affect every aspect of your life and close relationships in particular. Never before have relationships been as problematic and conflict ridden as they are now. As you may continue to pursue the goal of salvation through a relationship, you will be disillusioned again and again. But if you accept that the relationship is here to make you conscious instead of happy, then the relationship will offer you salvation, and you will be aligning yourself with the higher consciousness that wants to be born into this world. For those who hold to the old patterns, there will be increasing pain, violence, confusion, and madness.

—*Eckhart Tolle*, The Power of Now

When we have the opportunity to interact with others and they trigger an emotional response in us, we must be grateful! It is the very purpose for which we are in each other's lives. We are attracted to those people, events, and situations that will lead us to our highest potential at the level of the soul, always in all ways. We will keep attracting what we need to attract until we learn the lessons, and then we can move on. As we grow and become increasingly more aware on all levels, the emotional disruptions will eventually fade away. This is the path to enlightenment. This is how we tap into the Bliss Channel. This Bliss Channel is the cherry on top of the Journey to Joyful.

3. The third level is loving humanity through compassion.

The spirituality of Pranashama Yoga is discussed in Chapter 4.

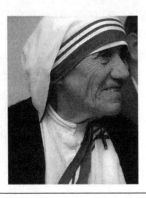

Mother Teresa, an embodiment of compassion.

Accessing the Bliss Channel

Bliss:

1. extreme happiness; ecstasy

2. the ecstasy of salvation; spiritual joy

Channel: AKA mediumship (also known as channeling), communication with spirit.

The Bliss Channel is the ability to access the state of supreme joy and happiness that we all seek in life. It is the direct connection to the Supreme Source, and I believe it is actually the highest state of the human experience. It is truly beyond description and can only be understood completely through direct experience. The Buddhists call this experience *Nirvana*. In Hinduism, this is known as *Samadhi*. Gnostic Christians refer to it as *Christ Consciousness*. Whatever your religious orientation, the experience transcends all systems of belief. In large part, I wrote this book specifically to help you access the Bliss Channel; and all of the tools, techniques, and guidance I offer are derived from the ancient traditions and teachings for this purpose.

In order for us to access the Bliss Channel, we must first become liberated from the emotional prison we have created for ourselves. Even as you read these words, observe your reactions. What arises for you in response to this concept? Perhaps an element of skepticism becomes present for you? Like, "That's not possible, Dashama!" or "That doesn't exist in Reality." It's okay if this is what arises for you, as all emotions have a time, a place, and a purpose.

Emotions exist for us to *feel* this self-created reality that we constructed around ourselves, referred to as Life. Emotion, sometimes referred to as *Energy in Motion*, guides us through our inner realms as we swim in this Ocean of Life. Like the natural pattern of a wave, the ocean can be turbulent one day and calm the next. Since our physical bodies contain more than 70 percent water, it is important that we embrace the water element of our emotions and dive into the vast dimensions of our emotional body. This enables us to understand both ourselves and others on a deeper level beyond judgment and duality. The *oneness* that results within and without transforms the feeling and experience of separateness, and unites us with the Supreme Source or the Divine Light of Love.

When we unite with Divine Love, we have direct access to the Bliss Channel. From my experience, this happens gradually for most people. We begin by having very short and brief glimpses into this seemingly hidden dimension of reality called Joy and Happiness. This often occurs during the times that we remember as peak experiences. Perhaps you recall an intimate interaction with a lover, a profound connection with nature, or the presence of joy you felt while gathered with your spiritual community.

I'll share with you a sweet story.

I have a special friend who began surfing at age three. He is amazing. He can go out in the big waves during a hurricane and feel at ease on his surfboard. One summer his family took him to Costa Rica for a month and he had the opportunity to surf every day on some of the most epic waves in the world. On day twenty-five of his magical month-long journey of connecting with the waves of Mother Nature in the way he loves most, a magical double rainbow appeared on either side of his tropical coastline. He fell into an ineffable state of bliss. With this story he shared the significance behind his Kaivalya Goddess tattoo, with its rainbows and ocean waves, that decorates his entire right shoulder. Knowing the meaning behind that story always makes me appreciate his colorful permanent body art even more. And for him, it serves as a constant reminder of that experience.

Connecting with Nature to Access the Bliss Channel

In my life, I have grown to understand that nature has the power of the universe or Supreme Source within it, and when we connect directly with her infinite power, we can easily drop into Bliss. We simply have to be open to receiving this blessing and willing to create space and time for these experiences to occur. This means connecting with nature on a regular basis—not just going out there and looking at the tree, but BEING with the TREE. Being IN the OCEAN. Climbing ON the ROCKS and MOUNTAINS. Appreciating nature in all of her magic and beauty. Allow yourself the gift of absorbing her pranic generosity and healing power.

Ask yourself the following questions:

What is my favorite way to connect with Mother Nature?

How do I *feel* when I am connected in that way?

The Meaning of *Namaste*: A True Story of Transformation

by Ryan Scott Seaman, Santa Monica, California

Namaste.

The embodiment of this ancient word is just one of countless transformations that the practice of yoga has brought to my life. Loosely translated, *namaste* means "The light in me bows to the light in you." This simple yet profound realization occurred, if only for a moment, in my first yoga class thirteen years ago. I was in my final semester at the University of Nebraska. On the surface I was living a life that closely resembled a dream. I had just returned from studying abroad in Australia, was about to graduate with honors, had a great job already lined up, and law school was on the horizon. Little did anyone know that for nearly three straight months I cried myself to sleep and could see no reason to continue living. I felt such a depth of despair that thoughts of suicide flooded the valley of my mind, and exercise was the only thing keeping me afloat.

One fateful Wednesday evening at the gym, I wandered upstairs to the aerobics room to do some quick stretching before I hit the weights. Six women were lined up on rectangular rubber mats. A seventh woman in her late fifties stood glowing at the front of the room. She smiled radiantly and asked me if I would like to join them. When I asked what they were doing, she smiled softly and uttered what would soon become the two most important syllables in my life: "Yoga." Some part of me (my Higher Self) said "yes," and before my ego could stop me, I became the seventh yogi in the class. An hour and a half later, lying on my back in my first ever *savasana*, tears streamed down my cheeks. These tears were different from what I had grown accustomed to in the months leading up to this moment. These tears were sourced not from the pain I'd been carrying but from the joy I thought was lost forever.

Yoga quickly became the foundation of a path to healing wounds I never knew existed. It was like a dam had been broken and an ocean of life force energy (*prana*) flooded through the deepest caverns of my mind, body, and heart. When I connected my movements with my breath, I unified parts of my self that for years prior had been fragmented. Yoga revealed light inside my darkest shadow, blessings within my most painful wounds, and the bliss of being alive at such an extraordinary time on this planet.

Today I practice yoga with great reverence for all life, to which I recognize I am infinitely connected. This connection helps me remember that we are all the manifestation of divine source energy, transcendent of religion. Paramahansa Yogananda said, "Everything else can wait, but our search for God cannot wait." Whenever I utter the word "*Namaste*" I'm reminded that I am God and so are you. Like Yogi Bhajan said, "If you can't see God in all, you can't see God at all."

CHAPTER 3

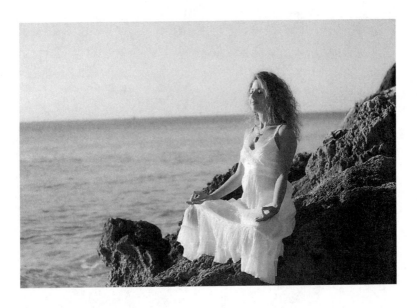

Taming the Monkey Mind

All that you are is a result of what you have thought.

—*The Buddha*

The Mind is where we cognize and give thought to all we experience. Before we even know how to use our body, our mind is already figuring out ways to survive in it. Our mind vibrates through the fifth (*Vishuddha*) and sixth (*Ajna*) chakra energy centers. Our fifth chakra resides in the throat center. When this energy center spirals freely, we express our truth and communicate free from inhibition or self-restraint. The sixth chakra resides in the third-eye center. When this energy center spirals freely, we access the inner vision of our higher mind and receive the guidance of our intuition.

When we're born, these channels flow freely with thoughts of divinity in the wonderment of all sense impressions. As we grow we develop our neural patterning in direct correspondence to our environment. Unfortunately, not all (and often very little) of what we see and experience cultivates a space for these energy centers to remain open. We instead develop conditioning that blocks how we perceive, limits what we're able to communicate, and closes us off altogether from our higher truth.

If we're born operating in a field of pure potentiality—unlimited and ever expanding—why do we often default into our negative habits and patterns, keeping us stuck and preventing us from accessing our highest potential? This is where *belief systems* and *patterns of identification* come into play.

From the moment we're born, and even during the nine months we spend in the womb, we are influenced by everything around us. We unavoidably perceive these influences as reality in order to create order out of the chaos of life. This is how our rational mind works. We're meaning-making machines. We formulate opinions, beliefs, and patterns to function in the construct of our society.

As infants we're sponges. We absorb the frequencies with which we're surrounded. We take on the imprints of what we witness. We mirror our masculine energy (left hemisphere of the brain) from our father, and our feminine energy (right hemisphere of the brain) from our mother. And thus we develop the assertive patterns of our father in harmonic opposition with the emotional receptors of our mother. Secondary levels of influence include siblings and others in our immediate environment, but the parents remain the primary influence in the development of our neural patterning, otherwise known as *limbic attractors*.

Early emotional experiences knit long-lasting patterns into the very fabric of the brain's neural networks.

—from A General Theory of Love *by Doctors Lewis, Amini, and Lannon*

Here's an obvious (albeit unpleasant) illustration of this principle in our world. A son born to the 41st President of the United States becomes the 43rd President. The literal dynamic of George Bush in this example is all too fitting. Not only do they share the same name, but they recycled the same war onto the canvas of this world. Out beyond the realms of political relevance (as if such a thing existed), a purely *objective* perspective recognizes the obvious paternal imprint lived out on life's stage.

In my personal reflection I recognize the process I underwent when my mother's addiction to alcohol vibrated through me. At a young age her vice became my vice. She also introduced me to yoga. Not only did she show me the shadow I would later reconcile, she introduced me to the practice I would need to do so. She guided me, just as all our teachers guide us when we can surrender our denial that this is exactly what we need in this moment. My mother remains my greatest teacher. In many ways her reflection allowed me to discover the purpose of my life. She opened in me both sides of the coin illustrated above. Her maternal imprint became the map through which I gained access to the channel of bliss available to us all *and* the sides of myself that need to be reconciled to sustain this connection.

We all have stories and we all live out the conditioning of our parents and society—until we step up and realize that the truth shall set us free. The key here is to take responsibility for how we work with the program that we know—in the *present moment*. We have two options here. We either reconcile the negative polarities or we remain in denial. I trust that if you're reading these words, you're in the camp that's on the path of reconciliation! In order to reconcile our conditioned mind we must undergo what's called *limbic revision*. This is where our relationships, whether with a teacher, a therapist, a lover or a friend, factor into the equation.

> When a limbic connection has established a neural pattern, it
> takes a limbic connection to revise it.
>
> —from A General Theory of Love *by Doctors Lewis, Amini,*
>   *and Lannon*

We encode new neural patterns through our myriad interactions with everyone we associate with. As we progress on our path of healing the wounded inner child—which in this case represents the unconscious aspect of ourselves that has attracted individuals into our lives that mirror what we're now ready to heal—we must take ownership of where we are and where we want to be. This hearkens back to what I mentioned earlier. We are the reflection of whomever we surround ourselves with. When you step into the arena of walking your truth, some of the people in your life will fall away, just as others will be attracted commensurate with your readiness to revise your antiquated belief systems and patterns of identification.

> Be not the slave of your own past—plunge into the sublime
> seas, dive deep, and swim far, so you shall come back with
> self-respect, with new power, with an advanced experience,
> that shall explain and overlook the old.
>
> —Ralph Waldo Emerson

Belief System

Belief System "Mental system consisting of interrelated items of assumptions, beliefs, ideas, and knowledge that an individual holds about anything concrete (person, group, object, etc.) or abstract (thoughts, theory, information, etc.). It comprises an individual's worldview and determines how he or she abstracts, filters, and structures information received from the world around. Also called cognitive system."

Identification

Identification A mental mechanism wherein the individual gains gratification, emotional support, or relief from anxiety by attributing to himself consciously or unconsciously the characteristics of another person or group.

In a world that operates under totally incongruent and oftentimes opposing belief systems, we're encountering an extraordinary combination of energy today on this planet and the charge is accelerating! On one side we have our outdated belief systems and identification with separation that naturally resist change. This is our conditioned mind. On the other side we have access to the Bliss Channel through which we have the opportunity to *create* with this increasing frequency. This is our higher mind. We're bridging the gap between the fifth and sixth chakras. When we do, the enormity of what we can create expands exponentially!

> Principles for the Development of a Complete Mind: Study the science of art. Study the art of science. Develop your senses— especially learn how to see. Realize that everything connects to everything else.
>
> —*Leonardo Da Vinci*

Look at our innovations in science and technology in the course of the last thirty years. The accelerated growth in the fields of biotechnology, nanotechnology, satellite communication, and silicon processing of information (just to name a few) is nearly incomprehensible! The same is true in art. Have you seen the work of Alex Gray? Did you watch the film *Avatar*? Extraordinary creations are flooding the planet from many artists.

When we resist the oppositional energies currently spiraling within us, we mirror this resistance around the planet through our perpetual wars and suffering in the world. *If we want more peace in the world, we must first begin within.* Until the opposition within our mind has been balanced, it will continue to manifest in the world.

Ideally by now we all recognize there's no question whether our thoughts create our reality. One thought has the creative power of the entire universe. What we think about we bring about. Life proves this time and again. If you sincerely observe your experience you will see this truth played out in all areas of your life. What you focus on grows, and what you avoid or ignore gets weaker and eventually dies. With this simple yet profound knowledge there must come understanding. If our thoughts are unlimited in potential, how is it that we are so prone to getting blocked from the ever-expansive nature of our creative flow? All too often we blame our circumstances, past and present, and spin off into a state of justifying, playing the tired role of victim. Get over it, whatever it is! There's no more room for denial at this stage in human evolution!

WE are the only things standing in our way, blocking the free flow of creative joy from streaming through our hearts and minds. Every time I run into the inevitable obstacle on my path, and my mind spirals into an ocean of fear, worry, or concern, I *stop* and *breathe.* I remember that the voices in my head have no connection to my true Self. This is the Monkey Mind.

In ancient yogic scriptures, the mind is often referred to as a "monkey" because it appears to have a will of its own and if we don't tame it, it will rule our lives. It will lead us from one poor choice to the next, driven by our ego's desire to satisfy our lower faculties of greed, lust, and power as a form of compensating for our unhealed wounds and unconscious emotional disharmony. You can see these tendencies in the actions of many world leaders, politicians, celebrities, and others who are in the public eye. You don't have to be publicly visible to suffer this mentality. It is not just some of us, but all of humanity that could use a little lesson in mind control. Not controlling the minds of others, but the control of one's own mind.

> Even the high Lamas of Tibet experience the ceaseless stream of thoughts running through our minds. The only difference is, we don't listen.
>
> —His Holiness the 14th Dalai Lama

The first step to transcending this ceaseless stream is to recognize that it exists. Simply **observe the thoughts as they arise.** Acknowledge the chaotic mental chatter that resounds throughout your mind from the moment you wake up until the final moment before you drift off to sleep at night. Meditate with the breath to quiet the mind. The use of *mantra* (see Appendix B) is one among many ways we can generate access to the Bliss Channel.

The second step is to journal what you observe. Simply **write down all and everything you think and feel.** And do so without judgment. Clear the mind of the ceaseless chatter. This will allow you to release yourself from identification with the content and open the energies of your throat chakra. From this energy center you communicate your personal truth. In this connection you can literally co-create your reality.

Take a moment here to explore what's spiraling through your mind.

Witness Consciousness

Utilizing a journal is a good way to gain mental clarity and practice witness consciousness. In a special notebook or simply on a sheet of paper, list the random stream of thoughts that are currently flowing through your Monkey Mind. Then detail what you feel is relevant from your list and what is mere mental chatter with no positive relevance in the here and now.

Are any of the thoughts you are working with in this journaling exercise recurring for you? In other words, do these circulate through your mind on a regular basis on other days? If so, write down those particular thoughts.

Which thoughts, if any, are positive and raising your conscious awareness in a way that is beneficial to your attitude, productivity, or happiness? Write them down.

Which ones are negative and possibly leading you to feel inferior, judgmental, attached, or any other condition that is not in alignment with your highest version of yourself? Write those thoughts down.

It should be pretty obvious by now what you're ready to let go of. Generally, when we observe our thoughts with total honesty and a desire to evolve, a beautiful thing happens: we see things crystal clear, just as they are. And we do so with no emotional connection to the events, circumstances, or people who are playing a role in this magical theatre of life. We are all here dancing together in a cosmic dance for the sheer pleasure of living life in these bodies. I honestly believe the purpose of life is to SIMPLY LIVE—joyously, unabashedly, openly, ecstatically, blissfully—and to share that radiant existence with others until they can feel that way too.

The third step is to **remember your true Self** beyond the existence of thoughts and the mechanism that generates them. This is where the power of intention comes into communion with the Third Eye. Here we access the Universal Mind (*Brahmandi*) and play with the cosmos to literally create our reality in alignment with our higher purpose.

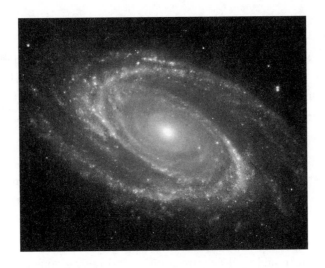

The only people for me are the mad ones, the ones who are mad to live, mad to talk, mad to be saved. The ones who never yawn or say a commonplace thing, but burn, burn, burn like fabulous yellow roman candles exploding like spiders across the stars.

—Jack Kerouac

Three Levels of Meditation

Level 1: Concentration (Dharana)—You focus to bring stillness to the mind. This can be done with Tratak candle-gazing meditation, during yoga practice while in *asanas*, or gazing at anything such as the sun, a *mandala*, etc. It is merely the quiet observation of the thoughts while focusing. This is the key. When we observe objectively the parade that is continuously marching in every direction of our mind, we can begin to see more clearly the root of our suffering. Buddhism calls this *samsara* or the *"wheel of suffering."* The Buddhist system of philosophy encourages control of the mind and emotions in order to minimize suffering and maximize happiness. I had the privilege to hear the Dalai Lama speak about the Four Noble Truths, which is fundamentally the Tibetan Buddhist key to moving toward enlightenment. At the core of these truths is the concept of non-attachment.

Level 2: Contemplation/Meditation (Dhyana)—At this level you are always in observation of your thoughts. You objectively and honestly assess the thoughts that arise within your consciousness and decide where they are arising from, whether they are serving you or acting as mere distractions, or just some cyclical pattern that is unnecessary and taking up valuable mental energy that could be better utilized elsewhere.

Level 3: Total Absorption (Samadhi)—In this state there are no discernable thoughts. We melt into the thoughtless, timeless space that occupies the other 99 percent of the universe. We merge with the Oneness from which we came and we unite with the Supreme Source. Typically in the unified thoughtless state we feel completely liberated and free. Love flows freely from our heart, and we feel connected to all that was, is, and ever will be. This is the goal of life: to live in that state, and to be able to operate in our very grounded lives here on Earth simultaneously. This is accessing the Bliss Channel.

> Create the highest, grandest vision possible for your life
> because you become what you believe.
>
> —Oprah Winfrey

Dreams Becoming Reality

First you must decide what you want . . . and write it down!

The universe will always give you what you ask for. The law of karma states that whatever you put out into the universe will come back to you—some say ten-fold! So deciding what you want is a good place to start.

After you decide upon your ideal vision for your life, then events and the specifics will fall into place for you. You will begin to attract the support and guidance you need to create your dreams and make them manifest into reality.

What is my highest vision for my life?

Write it down now. Be specific. If you already have a clear vision or even an idea of an interesting direction you'd like to explore in your life, write a short description of it in your notebook or on a sheet of paper.

Next write down what you would like your life to be like five, ten, or even twenty years from now.

My Personal Example

My life is a testament to the power of intention and visualization. I always knew I wanted to help people, but for many years I was lost as to what my life purpose could be. It was anguish trying to choose a major in college, because everything and nothing seemed interesting, and none of it seemed just right for me. I changed majors seven times until I realized it didn't really matter what degree I graduated with, since most people don't end up working in their field of study after college. That was comforting to know, to some extent, but unsettling at the same time.

I asked myself, why am I even going to college if I'm not going to use these years of study and accumulation of knowledge? At the time there didn't seem to be an alternative, and I had already begun the process so I continued on and found the most interesting and enjoyable major for me, which was Intercultural Communication and International Business. I knew I loved to travel. I loved people and learning about new cultures. It was always so intriguing to me to hear how differently we all live, yet we are all one big human family. I was even honored with the award "Student of the Year" for stumping my science professors with questions they had no answers for. I felt there must be a source of deeper wisdom that I could access.

I can remember a time when I was running on a trail behind the school and thinking, I wish I could just study energy! Where does it come from? How do some people have more than others? We are all energetic beings of vibrating molecules and atoms, so why don't they have a major we can study that teaches us how this all works? I wanted to know so I could tap into the infinite stream and even fantasized about learning to fly.

I later discovered Reiki energy healing, yoga, and Kundalini, the study of the control and manipulation of pranic energy systems, and I finally tasted the fruit of my seed question I had offered to the universe several years before. These studies were outside traditional university-level schooling, but they offered me exactly what I sought to study, so I dove in completely to my new interests.

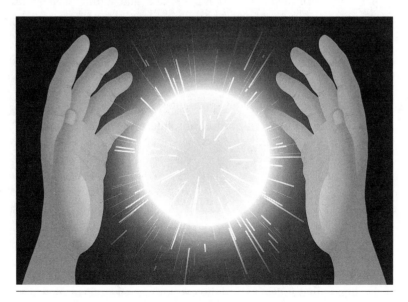

Energy healing

These types of occurrences are not rare. Often throughout my journey, I have had my questions answered for me, though not always immediately. This universe is not typically as instantly gratifying as we humans would love it to be. But sometimes it is. That is the magic of living in the mystery. You never know when the miracles will occur. You simply have to have faith and remain open to receive.

Keep asking the questions, though, and write them down. Thoughts put onto paper in the physical realm are far more powerful and creative in the world than those kept in the mind. They attract your answers much sooner. This is the reason for my second suggestion:

Ask the universe if there is anything blocking you from the attainment of your vision.

Challenges and obstacles will always arise to test us. Recently, when I was feeling overwhelmed with all I had on my plate, I asked myself, "Is there anything blocking me that may inhibit my ability to manifest my highest vision for my life RIGHT NOW?" and almost immediately the answer became clear. I heard this voice in my mind say, "You still have a personal lie that if you want things done right, you have to do them yourself." My lack of trust in others' ability to perform created a block in the flow of my creative output. With this realization I relinquished this personal lie and allocated specific tasks to others, trusting they would *exceed* my abilities. This proved absolutely true, right down to the completion of this book!

Karma

Life is a process of getting clear, neutralizing any negative karma so we may then transcend karma altogether to live in a state of pure potentiality and unbounded creativity. I believe it is in that state that we can truly align with our destiny and discover our *dharma* or life's work that we can be passionate about. If you are not familiar with karma, it is an essential aspect to understanding the how and why of life. The wise American philosopher Jim Rohn once told me, never ask why . . . like "why does the sun rise in the east and set in the west?" Who cares?! We can't change it; it's just the way it is. This is a valid way to look at life and can serve us on many occasions when we get trapped in the why and what-if mind games.

Let's explore that for a moment, though. I have come to understand that much of the "why" of our circumstance can be attributed to the principle of karma.

> **Karma:** (Hinduism and Buddhism) the effects of a person's actions that determine his destiny in his next incarnation; (Sanskrit: act, action, performance) the concept of "action" or "deed" in Indian religions understood as that which causes the entire cycle of cause and effect.

When we understand karma, we can begin to relax about the how and why of life. Instead of wondering why we had to go through some challenge in our life, we can attribute it to karmic debt that has carried over from a past life. Then we work in the present moment to release all karmic debt we may have accumulated. We do this by getting clear and by connecting to the Supreme Source through accessing the Bliss Channel.

> **Karma Yoga:** The word "karma" is derived from the Sanskrit Kri, meaning "to do." In its most basic sense "karma" simply means action, and "yoga" translates to union. Thus "Karma Yoga" literally translates to the path of "union through action." However, in Vedantic philosophy the word "karma" means both action and the effects of such action. Karma Yoga is described as a way of acting, thinking, and willing by which one orients oneself toward realiza- tion by acting in accordance with one's duty (dharma) without consideration of personal self-centered desires, likes, or dislikes. In

other words, acting without being attached to the fruits of one's deeds.

A few points about karma:

- It is believed possible to neutralize and even transcend negative or bad karma (both from this life and past lives), so everything you do in an effort to create good karma will help you to be reborn in a more favorable condition for your next life, in addition to improving the quality of your present life and the future for yourself and your family.
- There are many ways to build good karma in this life, and this book is full of options for you to work with right away.
- People with good karma tend to have an easier time creating what they want in life and attracting positive experiences.
- Often you are blessing others in your pursuit of good karma, which is the very essence of the practice, and by being a blessing to others, you will also be blessed richly in return by the law of giving and receiving. When you give, you automatically receive and the cycle is unending.
- Although there may be more power in selfless service on a universal level, any good deeds are acknowledged by the energy of the universe and set the wheels in motion for you to participate in the giving and receiving process. Begin wherever you are, and with time, the giving will be so rewarding that you won't even think of potential for receiving, as it is inherently built into the process.

The ultimate experience of giving is to make what might otherwise seem like work into something to enjoy and look forward to. When we perform our Karma Yoga actions from a space of obligation to give, act, or do something, we limit our ability to experience the greatest benefit of the action—which is complete JOY! For people who give with an open willing heart, it is not work; it is the best possible use of their time. For people who drag their feet at the thought of volunteer work, it is heavy and unbearable. You decide which you would prefer to embark upon and set your mind and heart in advance. It is you who will ultimately feel the blessings if you choose love and willingness.

This principle is invaluable to teach to children. Possibly you have learned your behavior in relationship to giving and receiving from your parents.

According to many ancient teachings, karma determines your birth to a certain extent. If you have some unresolved karma from past lives, you may be born into a family that will help facilitate the healing of those issues on a soul level, so you may move on to better life circumstances beginning immediately.

I chose my birth.

In large part, I believe my soul chose to be born into the family I was born into because it offered the best possible chance to evolve rapidly. My soul knew it had to be strong to do the work I am here to do in this life, so I was faced with some very challenging circumstances early on. Watching the deterioration of my mother's health was not easy, but it helped me to transcend any fear of death and to release my attachment to people as well. She taught me many positive things while she was alive, such as yoga, healthy eating, and how to live with a very light carbon footprint. These were priceless life lessons for which I am eternally grateful.

Some people's karma is so inspiring it is noteworthy.

Allow me to illustrate with a living example. We're blessed to listen to Anoushka Shankar, daughter of the sitar maestro Ravi Shankar, create mystical rhythms and melodies from the instrument her father mastered. It's as though she's channeling bliss through every chord she strokes. Anoushka reflects the pure essence that a child picks up from a parent in their developmental years. When we allow ourselves to open

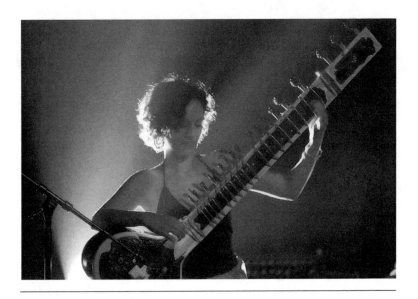

Anoushka Shankar

with her to that channel of bliss inside ourselves, we open to receiving love through every octave of creation. Not knowing her personal challenges, I can only imagine she must have accumulated great karma to be born unto a family where her father is a living master and spiritual guru. This is a beautiful example of a blessed life we can aspire to create for ourselves both now and in future incarnations.

On the other end of the spectrum, children who are born into an unhealthy family and/or environment often grow up with a skewed perspective of reality. Modeling the adults and others around them, they often learn how to operate in a very unhealthy and unfulfilling way. Parents who lacked nurturing environments as they were growing up tend to offer the same to their offspring. Poor dietary habits including fast food, junk food, and highly processed foods are most commonly passed on from one generation to the next. This is a form of unconscious neglect that is all too common in our world today. Parents using and abusing drugs, alcohol, and tobacco offer poor role models to their growing children. Adults struggling with health concerns, sickness, obesity, and disease demonstrate to children that this is common and to be expected as part of their "genetic" code. We believe what we see, and what we see conditions our mind. And round and round we go, until we recognize. . . .

> The thinking mind is a wonderful servant, but a terrible master.
>
> —*Swami Vivekananda*

Controlling Our Mind

If only all people knew, as I am sharing with you now, that all of the above-mentioned factors are variables in the continuum of our life experience and that we have the ability to take control of this all—mastering our health, well-being, and ultimately the entire destiny of our life.

Knowing this, and seeing people take control of their destiny and reformulate their perceptions and experience of reality, is motivation enough to get the word out. Once you understand this fundamental principle of life, you can no longer stand by and allow people to drown in their poor habits and negative and limiting beliefs, and watch them deteriorate in front of you. You have to reach out a hand, throw them a life jacket, and welcome them into the family of Life. But before we can help others, we must first help ourselves. When we're a shining example of the potential of human evolution, we inspire others to want to change.

> You cannot change people, but they can change themselves.
>
> —*Jim Rohn*

Chitta Vritti Nirodha—calming the mental fluctuations of the mind. All great yogis will tell you that that is the key to enlightenment. In that space of mental clarity, all possibilities exist. Unbounded creativity, infinite potential, and bliss reside beyond the mental chatter.

This is achieved in many ways. You can sit still in lotus position with eyes closed or trance dance to music that moves the room and rocks your soul. I'm here to share with you all of this. There's no "one size fits all" way to attaining enlightenment. Not to mention, it's much more fun to try new things! If you keep it interesting you will stick to your path. As you do, you will see all the hours of practice (*sadhana*) manifesting in the person you are becoming. Your radiant inner being will begin to shine brighter and ever more luminescent every day.

Mindset

What makes the difference between an Olympic athlete and someone who struggles to get off the couch? While genetics certainly factor into the equation, *much of our current health and happiness come down to lifestyle choices, mindset, and attitude.* You determine the course of your path with each decision you make.

Do you choose to eat Doritos and nacho cheese while watching Monday night football, or do you eat celery sticks dipped in organic raw hummus while listening to upbeat music and planning your sunset hike through the forest or your next yoga session?

This is just one example, but each day you are faced with hundreds of similar decisions, each seemingly insignificant, but when we combine the accumulated effect of these lifestyle choices over time, we begin to see our choices showing up in our body and in our life. We see the sum total of those nachos in our thighs and hips, the quart of ice cream in our lower belly, and the deep-fried chicken wings with extra blue cheese bursting the seams of our favorite pair of jeans.

It's up to you. Instead of unconsciously consuming empty calories, take a deep breath. Check in with why you're eating what you're eating. What emotions are you covering up and excusing through the justification of your conditioned mind? *Find the truth and the truth will set you free.*

We base our lives on seeking happiness and avoiding suffering, but the best thing we can do for ourselves—and for the planet—is to turn this whole way of thinking upside down.

—Pema Chodron, Buddhist meditation teacher

Tibetan Buddhism uses the term shenpa to describe a profoundly simple technique for mental and emotional control. This term has such elaborate meaning, it's difficult to describe in English. Essentially it refers to the hook or trigger that takes your mind from a state of relaxed thoughts drifting in and out, to an emotionally charged spiral of thoughts that can often spin out of control.

The good news: knowing about shenpa makes us more compassionate toward others. We can acknowledge that they are experiencing this very same chaos inside their minds too! We are not alone in this quirky human experience, after all!

If a shenpa is a trigger or a hook, it can be a thought that drives you to reach for food and numb the frazzled state of your mind that's actually preventing you from feeling a deeper core emotion. This is when overconsumption often occurs for most people. While a person sits there eating unconsciously, for that short period of time, they don't have to think or feel what's really underneath.

So, you may be wondering, how do we get rid of shenpa?

The truth is, these triggers don't go away easily. Our conditioned mind has been developed over the duration of our lives, and so revising it to harmonize with our intuitive mind won't occur overnight. The key is awareness. If you recognize them each time they are activated, by shining the light of awareness on them, they will begin to grow dimmer and dimmer. Then finally, they won't have such an effect on you.

Here are a few questions to ask yourself that may help you figure out what your shenpas are and how you can begin to gain some control over them.

1. Name one thing (or several if you are really ready to go in deep) that triggers or brings an emotional response into your mind and entire body—that once you feel it, it is difficult to shake or release the emotion. (This can be negative or positive; although for practicality's sake, we are really only concerned with the negative ones that make us behave rashly or rudely, with anger or irritation, etc.)

   An example may be thoughts of a past relationship that didn't work out and ended painfully; or a situation where you felt guilty for something and never got a chance for reconciliation; a person (such as your boss) that you feel treats you with disrespect or unfairness; or an event that still brings a huge emotional response like the death of a loved one, etc.

2. Now, recognizing the *shenpa*, make it a practice to notice when something triggers it for you. All you do is simply acknowledge: "That's a *shenpa*." And then just let the thoughts and emotions go. If you can't let it go, breathe with it, deep breaths into your heart until it's gone.

   A lot of times we pretend that nothing is wrong. This is often unsuccessful when you're with someone who knows you well. A friend, spouse, or partner will notice the obvious shift in your energy and attitude.

   This is a mindfulness meditation and a daily expansion of your willingness to live your life as a compassionate and loving individual. This is your internal medicine.

Bull in a China Shop: A True Transformation Story

by Sharla Patrick, NC

For the past eight or so years I have noticed a common theme in my life—stress. I've often been called a "bull in a china shop" or "Tasmanian devil," and I find that it's hard for me to slow down.

That all changed November 2008 when I was introduced to the beautiful practice of yoga at an amazing retreat I attended. I went to the beach early morning with a big towel in hand and no clue how yoga would transform my life.

I could feel the cool sand beneath my feet as I stepped onto my towel; I could feel the vibration of the waves crashing against the shore. We began class in a seated position while just focusing on our breath, and boy did I start to connect with Spirit and the world around me in that very instant. As I stared at the ocean and felt the wind on my face, I felt like an infant experiencing these things for the first time ever.

Each pose we did was challenging yet so invigorating. To begin this process really slowed down what often seems to be a crazy whirlwind of life. I felt my body. I was communicating with my body and enjoyed every minute of this practice.

I was so enthralled with these feelings that I started a regular yoga practice from that point on. In general I practice at home about three to five times a week. I have taken a 30-Day Yoga Challenge with the beautiful soul Dashama Konah and felt one of the biggest shifts in my life—physically, mentally, and spiritually.

My physical body was so much more flexible. Mentally I felt that I was more solution-oriented than problem-focused; I also felt more calmness in my life during and after the Challenge. In addition, I grew spiritually in my everyday life because of the 30-day "journey" I went on.

Yoga has in every way given me more balance to an often chaotic and stressed life. I find solace in my yoga practice. Now instead of feeling like a "Tasmanian devil" or "bull in a china shop," I feel peace like never before and I love it! What a better place to operate from.

CHAPTER 4

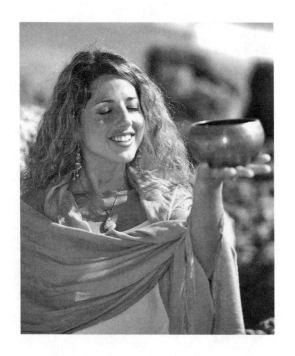

Spiritual Liberation

Are You Ready to Break Free?

I feel strongly that my life is to be used as an example of what
can be done.

—Oprah Winfrey

Throughout this book, I have interwoven the spirituality of Pranashama
Yoga. Through the stories, techniques, and philosophy, I hope you have
begun to grasp the essence of the teachings I am sharing. If it hasn't
been clear up until now, I will further illustrate the basis from which
all of this is intended to lead you toward a liberated state of enlightened
joy and bliss.

Samadhi or enlightenment is the ultimate goal of the Eight Limbs of
Yoga. It is characterized by the state of ecstasy and the feeling that you
and the universe are one. It is a state of peace and completion, awareness
and compassion with detachment.

When I first read the Buddhist teachings of the Dalai Lama, especially
those regarding the philosophy that "all life is suffering," I fell into a
deep depression. I thought, what is the point then? If we are here simply
in suffering and there is no way around it, why even live? I later read a
book titled The Yoga Vasistha* that helped to clarify this area of ambiguity.

In The Yoga Vasistha, the young prince in the book experiences something similar to what I went through, although from a very different
perspective. He grew up in a castle amongst royalty. He never left the
castle grounds where he was raised. And the royal spiritual advisor,
named Visthistha, was there throughout to provide answers when the
prince questioned the purpose of life and other philosophical ponder-
ings. One day the prince decided he must see the world and embarked
upon a two-year tour through the countryside. During his travels he
saw the deepest despair and poverty, beyond his wildest imagination.

* Christopher Key Chapple and Swami Venkatesananda, The Concise Yoga Vasistha (Albany:
State University of New York Press, 1984).

Upon returning to the castle, he could not eat. He could not continue living in the same lavish way he had been so accustomed to. He fell into the same deep depression that I did.

So what do we do?

When I read this I could completely relate, but at the same time, I was looking for answers! I wanted to know, well . . . what do we do?

I was looking for the happy ending and rainbows. It was through a sincere process of inner seeking and meditation that I pulled out of the depression (in addition to extensive yoga practice, physical exercise, and positive affirmations).

The real key for me was to have my deep longing for the Truth revealed to me. And this occurred through the study and practice of Tantra Yoga, *Seva*, and the *Bodhichitta* path. Prior to these discoveries, I had studied conceptual principles and practices that should eventually lead to some esoteric experience of "enlightenment." This all seemed so impractical that I just couldn't get very interested in any of them. I had felt confined by the rules in the Bible, Torah, and Koran. Each offered brilliant wisdom that could be gleaned, but the parameters within which they suggested I was "allowed" to operate "according to the word of God" were very strict and limited.

When I truly realized the limitless and ever-expanding Truth of my Soul, a tremendous weight was lifted from my shoulders and out of my heart.

I was looking for something I could FEEL, TASTE, EXPERIENCE, and know as REAL-LIFE BLISS. And one of the first ways in which I touched upon it was through the teachings of Kundalini Tantra as well as the Transformation of Desire/Buddhist Tantra and the timeless classic, the Bhagavad Gita.* These three texts brought me out of my depression, along with providing a great deal of joy and newfound excitement about the yogic path!

*Sri Swami Satchidananda, *The Living Gita: The Complete Bhagavad Gita, a Commentary for Modern Readers* (Yogaville, Va.: Integral Yoga Publications, 1988).

Tantra Yoga and True Liberation

Tantra: a set of spiritual practices and ritual forms of worship that aim toward liberation from ignorance and achieving a rebirth. These beliefs and practices work from the principle that the universe we experience is nothing other than the concrete manifestation of the divine energy of the Supreme Source that creates and maintains that universe. Tantra seeks to ritually appropriate and channel that energy, within the human microcosm, in creative and emancipatory ways.

Out beyond ides of wrong doing and right doing, there is a field. I'll meet you there. . . .

—Rumi, *twelfth-century Sufi mystical poet*

Most people in Western society associate Tantra with sex. This is so inaccurate and limited in its perspective. Tantra is a path that leads to complete union with the Supreme Source. The teachings vary based upon the lineage, just like all yoga paths. The Buddhist Tantra teachings have illuminated my path in the most profound way, and for that reason, I will share the teachings with you. Following is a brief discussion of some of the most important aspects of the path.

It is important to know that *bliss is accessible primarily through the heart center and the experience of compassion.*

Being in service to humanity opens the portal for bliss, when we are aligned with our highest potential and purpose, doing the work we have come to Earth to do. There are many ways in which to attain this state of bliss, and however you get there, it is the experience of being there that is the important part. When we access the highest heights at least once, it is much easier to find our way back. I like to call it "flashbacks to bliss."

I have accessed this state of bliss many times in many ways. It has blossomed in my heart during peak experiences like standing upon the top of Half Dome (a granite monolith in Yosemite Valley) after hiking for fourteen hours up 10,000 feet and being able to see down into the valley directly below me and all around as far as the neighboring state. I have also accessed this bliss while in communion with Mother Nature and people very near and dear to me. Chanting sacred *mantras* is a way to access bliss, and so is the practice of the Thai Yoga Prana Flow that I teach. Most profound of all, however, is the feeling that I experience when I offer my heart and soul to others who will benefit from my energy and love.

Enlightenment Is Bliss

Through all my practices and studies I've come to recognize enlightenment as synonymous with bliss. In a life full of ironies, it feels all too appropriate that the same esoteric concept that turned me away from the ancient teachings brought me back from depression and helped to solidify my commitment to this path.

It didn't end there. Life was not roses and bliss every minute after that, trust me. It rarely ever is.

When you first discover the Truth of Existence, it is usually just a glimpse. The Supreme Source is offering this expanded awareness as bait to keep us on the path. It happens over and over again. Just when I feel like giving up and throwing in the hat on the whole process of becoming clear light (enlightenment), the Universe presents something so unmistakably obvious that I am reminded that it is all worthwhile and I am on the right track.

To remain disciplined and have faith are the daily tests.

I was at a gathering in Miami with Alex and Allison Grey, both regarded as two of the most enlightened visionary artists of our time. Something Alex said really stuck with me when I asked him, "What inspires you to get out the paintbrushes and canvas, and pour your heart and soul into a creative work of art?" He responded, "Allison. She'll ask me, have you painted anything today?" And it was really that simple. So, as the old Zen proverb goes:

Before enlightenment chop wood and carry water.
After enlightenment, chop wood and carry water.

—Wu Li

So, when we reach enlightenment, we still have to work?

The concept of work is a perception of the mind. We learn at a very young age the societal difference between work and play. Work is something we have to do, but don't want to do. Play is the opposite. We grow up resisting work and longing to play more. This dissonance between what we have and what we want creates great suffering—mostly psychologically. But when we embrace suffering on any level, as we learned in Chapter 2, the emotional experience affects us on all levels. And the source of the deepest suffering is our illusion of being separate from the Creator.

It is the deepest pain we can inflict upon ourselves. At the same time—and here is the really important key—**separation is all an illusion.**

We create this whole story that plays out in these dramas and attracts situations to us that make us believe we are separated from the Supreme Source.

The Truth is: We are NEVER SEPARATE.

That is the cosmic joke. The incredible parody is that we are so deeply involved in the story lines that we miss the "bigger picture" that I spoke about earlier.

If we would, even just for one moment, step into the Truth of who we are, beyond the self and ego-created version of who we are that is really experiencing these tremendously painful life situations, we will step into a state of unbelievably expanded awareness, bliss, and joy.

We are addicted to our own suffering. This is the fundamental disease of our time. Not cancer, not AIDS, or any one specific disease, as most people might assume. It is a psychological fact that *the human mind prefers misery over change!*

The number-one addiction and cause of all death is this addiction to suffering.

We live in fear of accessing total expansive awareness and bliss. So we create a whole world and lifetimes of melodrama to support our belief system and feed our ego. Our ego loves to be right. It loves to know it is doing the best it can and that if things are out of harmony, it is because we are somehow the victims of someone or something.

According to the ego, we are perfect and at the same time we are so worthless that we do not deserve to be united with God. This is the real devil. Not some mythological character from the Bible wearing a sinister red cape with blood-stained horns growing out of his head. That is for storybooks and fairy tales.

The real devil is that which holds the veil of illusion, called *Maya* in Sanskrit. It keeps us from seeing the truth of who we are. And seeing it this way, it is our goal to break free from the chains that have been holding us captive for so long and enter entirely into the light, leaving the darkness and illusion of separation far behind, like a bad dream or an old worn memory that doesn't affect you anymore.

You are FREE. You are ALIVE.

You are radiantly, vibrantly, joyfully, and blissfully more alive that you may have ever imagined possible. And even by that description I am limited in my ability to describe who you really are. It must be FELT. It is beyond thoughts. Beyond words. Beyond physical form.

> Knowing eternity makes one comprehensive; comprehension makes one broadminded; breadth of vision brings nobility; nobility is like heaven.
>
> —Lao-Tzu

How do we access this awareness? Well, according to Gangaji and Allan Watts, two great spiritual teachers from the twentieth century, we can access this at any moment when we simply drop the veil. **Let it all go.** Let go of the idea that it is going to be a lot of work. Let go of that idea that we need to even follow a path, such as yoga or Buddhism. I teach the path to freedom, liberation, and BLISS. You may have noticed, the tools and techniques I offer are not all from the traditional yogic lineages. And there are a few yogic lineages that I merge, incorporating what I find to be the more effective and beneficial aspects of each, while integrating techniques from internal and external martial arts, Chinese Medicine, Taoism, Tantra, Reiki, Eating Prana, and Living on Light.

I've noticed over the years that people resist the ideas of "therapy" and "healing." Sort of like, "If I'm not physically injured, then I don't need *healing or therapy.*" These two often have a negative connotation attached to them; I would like to clarify these two terms so there is no confusion or ambiguity.

Everyone on this path to enlightenment needs healing on some level.

We use healing techniques to clear ourselves from our past, so we can live more fully in the present. Everyone has inner-child issues; we all have past-life karma we're dealing with. It's only the ego that prevents us from admitting this and being open to the process.

Stop, right now, and be honest. Is this true for you? Thank you.

The term "therapy" actually describes anything you do to heal yourself. So everything can fall into this category. Yoga, massage, talk therapy, laughter therapy, music therapy, etc. The methods are plentiful. It is important that we take responsibility for our needs free from our ego's pride and fear of humiliation. This is the first step in letting the stiffness go and becoming OPEN, which is synonymous with CLEAR, LIGHT, ENLIGHTENED, or BLISSFUL.

Language is so interesting. Two people can have a conversation in the same language and completely miss each other's point. The reason

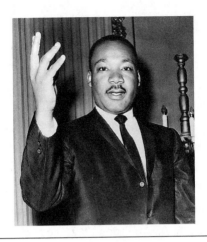

Dr. Martin Luther King Jr.

for this is that we all place such variable meanings upon these words, which, from our narrow perspective, we believe are universally understood and definitive. This is never the case. Truly effective communicators know this and make sure to relate to each other in as many ways as possible during the process of communication, to ensure their message is being received well and as accurately as possible.

If you are interested in being happy and successful in life, it is of paramount importance that you learn to be an excellent, compassionate communicator who can relate to a variety of people. It is not necessarily easy, but it is a highly rewarding endeavor worthy of your efforts.

Love Is My Religion

I drank the wine of which the soul is its vessel. Its ecstasy has stolen my intellect away. A light came and kindled a flame in the depth of my soul. A light so radiant that the sun orbits around it like a butterfly.

—Rumi, *twelfth-century Sufi mystical poet*

When people ask me if yoga is a religion, I smile and answer *not at all*. Although there are certain styles and schools of yoga that embrace and interweave their own religious views, Pranashama Yoga embraces all views while honoring Love and Unity above all else. As you may have noticed, I often quote masters, saints, and enlightened people throughout this book and other teachings. I do this to illustrate the point that they are all brilliant and connected deeply to the Supreme Source. They each have their own spin on this life experience, and much of what they offer is valid and applicable, even after thousands of years.

Truth is Timeless. Love is Eternal. Bliss is Infinite.
We are All One. United at the Supreme Source.

Bodhichitta and the Gateway between Heaven and Earth

Heaven is a mental construct we have created, adopted from the teachings of the Bible and other traditions, to express the infinite beyond this world of form. Even if you don't believe in heaven or hell, it is a good word that we can use to reference the Space Beyond our life on Earth that is Perfect, Blissful, and Everlasting. Whatever that place is for you is perfect. It lives eternally within our hearts.

The heart center is the gateway between heaven and earth, spiritual and physical realms, and the human experience of embodying the essence of Love and Oneness with other beings on Earth and beyond. Through the heart we are able to access the deepest levels of compassion, joy, and bliss. The heart chakra acts as the bridge between the lower chakras that represent life and the upper chakras that represent spirit. When we are disconnected from our heart center, we are blocked from receiving the divine healing and transformative transmissions from the Supreme Source and grounding them here on Earth. This is the key to accessing our highest human potential.

May the Lord continually bless you with heaven's blessings as well as with human joys.

—*Psalms* 128:5

Bodhichitta is the wish to attain complete enlightenment in order to be of benefit to all sentient beings trapped in cyclic existence (Samsara) who have not yet reached enlightenment. One who has *bodhichitta* as the primary motivation for all of his or her activities is called a *bodhisattva*. *Bodhi* means "awakening" or "enlightenment."" *Chitta* is derived from the Sanskrit root *chit* and denotes "that which is conscious"—mind or consciousness. *Bodhichitta* may be translated as "awakening mind" or "mind of enlightenment." *Bodhichitta* may also be defined as the union of compassion and wisdom. This is a development of the concept of luminous mind.

Bodhichitta may be viewed as having different levels: one useful classification is that given by Patrul Rinpoche in his *Words of My Perfect Teacher*. He states that the lowest level is the way of the King, who primarily

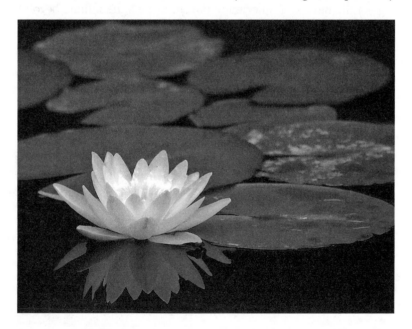

seeks his own benefit but who recognizes that his benefit depends crucially on that of his kingdom and his subjects. The middle level is the path of the boatman, who ferries his passengers across the river and simultaneously, of course, ferries himself as well. The highest level is that of the shepherd, who makes sure that all his sheep arrive safely ahead of him and places their welfare above his own.

Bodhisattva

Bodhisattva (Buddhist philosophy): one whose essence is enlightenment.

My Personal Example

There came a time in my life when I realized I wanted nothing more than to be of service to humanity. This came to me full force through my experience with the Christian church. I had an experience with Jesus that moved me in such a way that I was forever changed. My heart was burst open and I felt like I was bleeding love. I felt deeply within my soul that I wanted to be of service to humanity with my life. I tried doing various jobs and businesses, but inevitably I felt unhappy, since the primary purpose for most of them was to make money. That was not nourishing to my soul.

I desired to do something that was meaningful, that would be of service to humanity in the greatest way possible, and that I could enjoy. Through the teaching of yoga and the many creative and humanitarian avenues, I am able to express my soul's voice—I am content. Whether it is through writing books, teaching classes, workshops, and retreats, producing and creating videos and other instructional material, organizing charitable events, trance dances, and yoga fire-dancing performances, I have so many outlets for my abundant creativity that I am never bored. And best of all, I know I am helping people transform their lives, which is the most rewarding feeling in existence.

I don't know what your destiny will be, but one thing I know: the only ones among you who will be truly happy are those who have sought and found how to serve.

—*Albert Schweitzer*

Seva

Seva is "selfless service" in Sanskrit. This is another way to offer your time and efforts for the good of humanity. This is more of an action and does not so much refer to a life path. That is the fundamental difference between *seva* and *bodhichitta*. There are many *seva* projects that may be available for you to participate in if you wish to offer your time, energy, or resources to help others for a good cause. One example is the Yoga for Foster Kids (and Orphans) foundation that I created. I am also a partner with National Yoga Month and their Yoga Health Foundation that raises money to bring yoga into public schools everywhere. A portion of all profits from the 30-Day Yoga Challenge and all other sources is used to fund both of those non-profit philanthropic organizations.

Finding Your Life Purpose

At the center of your being, you know who you are and you know what you want.

—*Lao-Tzu*

I feel incredibly grateful to have found my life purpose so early in life. Thanks to the abundance of technology and information available to us, it is much easier to explore and discover your life purpose than ever before.

The how-to guides are all available; the tools and techniques are readily offered, and you merely have to trust the guiding voice of your intuition. It will rarely steer you wrong. I've known many people who have been divinely guided to pick up a book in a bookstore and it

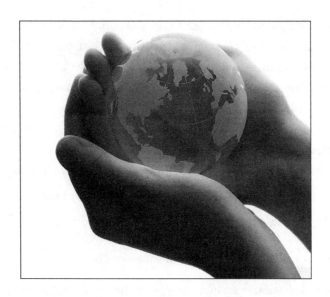

changed the entire course of their life for the better. You will be in the right place at the right time and you merely have to be awake and alert to the signs and signals being transmitted to you.

Who am I and why am I here?

This question is on everyone's mind. If it's not on yours yet, it will be at one point in your life. You will find yourself in a place where you have spent a great deal of time DOING and GOING and LIVING, but you question what is the purpose of all of this? What am I best suited to offer this world, during this lifetime? These questions are the miracle seeds that will grow into the fruit that nourishes you, providing you with all of the answers.

According to the Bible, Jesus said, "Ask and you shall receive." From this you may deduce that you won't receive until you ask. So first ask the Universe to provide you with guidance in finding your life's purpose.

Why do some people get things they don't ask for?

We are always asking for something at some level, whether it is externally, verbally, or internally, at the level of the subconscious mind. We are constantly requesting from the universe that we be given something—answers to prayers, physical and non-physical things of all sorts.

This is why meditation is so powerful. During the practice of meditation we are able to stop all activity and witness the internal dialogue. In doing this, we explore our hidden and overt desires and dreams. It will also ideally lead us to discovering our life purpose and ultimately our *dharma*.

Dharma means one's righteous duty, method, or any virtuous path.

If you really want to discover your life purpose, a wonderful technique is to sit in quiet meditation and visualize the movie of your ideal life.

Try journaling the answers to the questions below:

If you had all the money in the world, all the free time, and were supported completely in all ways, what would you do with your time?

What do you enjoy doing?

With so many subcultures of people it is first necessary to see where you feel you best fit in. And don't worry if you don't feel like you fit in somewhere right away. It will come to you over time as you explore more deeply who you are and why you are here.

What type of people do you admire and love to spend time with? Intellectual people? Those who focus on service to others? People who are highly into the health and well-being of the physical body?

Write down the limitations you feel are preventing you from living the life of your dreams. Please be specific and honest (e.g. money, your appearance, low self-esteem, etc).

Imagine you are looking at yourself from an outside perspective, as the observer. Write down a list of traits that would best describe you (e.g. fun, adventurous, friendly, shy, health-conscious, intelligent, organized, etc.).

How would you like to be remembered when you're gone? (Examples: for what you created; for what you gave; for how you treated others, etc.)

This visualization practice is tremendously powerful. Simply by writing these ideas down, you are already putting them out there into the universe. In our society, we are programmed from day one to believe we are limited in so many ways. Our government, teachers, parents, and associates all encourage us to follow a system and do what everyone else does. This generally does not lead you to unveiling your ultimate dreams and goals, however.

You will never live life beyond your wildest expectations until you first have some wild expectations!

Whether you would like to be in a happy relationship and raise your children in peace and harmony, or you would like to be financially independent and travel the world snowboarding on the highest mountain peaks, or you wish to serve the poor and destitute as a global missionary, you have the capacity to live your dreams in this lifetime. The key is to do it in service to others. That's what makes the difference between living a spiritual life and one devoid of true depth and meaning.

It is important to do what you love, as that will lead you to the success and happiness you seek. I have known many people who create businesses, careers, and *dharmas* out of their hobbies. I have met people who make successful businesses that they thoroughly enjoy out of their passion for wedding planning, gift basket creation, doggie watching, interior design, fashion design, kite boarding, surfing, yoga teaching, and many other fun and creative jobs. I have also known people to attract their dream relationship purely by writing down all the qualities they desire in a mate, and that person magically appears in their life as if sent from a higher source who could read minds!

Writing it down is the key.

One New Year I wrote a list of goals and dreams. I was lofty and realistic simultaneously. I put specific financial, personal, physical, relational goals on the list. Then I lost the list and couldn't find it for eight months. When I finally found it, I had accomplished or attracted more than half of the items without even thinking about it. If I'd have had it accessible to read over, I know I would have been able to cross off even more of these goals.

Be patient—sometimes it takes a little while. Sometimes what you want doesn't come right away because you simply are not ready to receive it yet. This is very common. You want something but know you really need to grow a bit more before you'll be able to handle the fullness of the blessing you are asking to receive. The universe is not always on the same time schedule as we would like!

What is important is that you decide *what* you love and want in your life, and then the *how* will come to you. You will begin to attract the people, resources, and information you need to move in that direction. The universe will always support whichever path you put thought into. *There are no right or wrong paths in life.* There are only innumerable opportunities to experience life in its fullness and richness, growing and learning all along the way.

Be careful of limitation thinking. When the thoughts of "I can't," "impossible," "not me" come into your mind, let them go right away. These are the seeds of disaster and the barriers to your success. Remember that the opposite thought waves exist and ride those! "Of course I can," "Absolutely," "Yes, me!" Be mindful of what you're thinking and unhook from the negative patterns. You are consciously and unconsciously creating and attracting everything in your life at all times.

Faith is the strength by which a shattered world shall emerge
into the light.

—*Helen Keller*

Gratitude and Appreciation

Gratitude: a feeling of thankfulness and appreciation.

Appreciation: recognition of the quality, value, significance, or magnitude of people and things.

This book would not be complete without mentioning the importance and significance of gratitude and appreciation. These are two of life's most precious gifts. When we express and experience gratitude and appreciation, we open the floodgates of love in our hearts and allow the true spiritual essence of life to shine through us. Every moment contains a hundred opportunities to be grateful and appreciate what IS. Regardless of whether we think what we are currently experiencing is good or bad, beyond the limited scope of our perspective, we must have faith that everything is for the highest good. And with that mindset, we have no other choice than to be extremely grateful for the blessings that we are given. Be grateful for the people who are put in your life to illuminate your strengths and weaknesses. Be grateful for your circumstances, knowing that you have attracted and created everything you are experiencing in your life right now. And most of all, be grateful for the awareness that you can change your circumstances, as long as you are willing to change your mindset.

Take this opportunity to write down a list of things you are grateful for right now.

As soon as possible, call, write, or make an appointment to see the people on this list and tell them how grateful you are. Show your appreciation, even if it is just a hug or a thoughtful note. If possible, do something for them. Trust me, this goes a long way.

There are some cultures that make it customary never to visit someone without bringing something to offer. It doesn't have to be much. It can be a flower, a card, or just a blessing you say or feel in your heart. Just make it a habit to share and give whenever possible, and you will be unlocking the gates for blessings and appreciation to flow freely within your own life as well.

Stay Inspired and Live with Passion!

Inspiration: the act or power of exercising an elevating or stimulating influence upon the intellect or emotions; the result of such influence which quickens or stimulates, such as the inspiration of occasion, of art, etc. Also, inhalation, the act of taking a breath.

So we have come full circle back to the breath, the most vitally essential aspect to our existence, without which life would cease. Pranashama Vinyasa Yoga is the bridge that connects your body with your spirit through your breath. And it is the daily practice that serves as the daily inspiration.

We all need to be inspired, to continue to create, to move forward with passion and excitement about life. It is true that we must be content with the simplicity of life, so it isn't constant stimulus and excitement that I am referring to. It is that link to the joy, bliss, and compassion that we need to stay inspired for. And that comes in many forms.

Beauty of whatever kind, in its supreme development,
invariably excites the sensitive soul to tears.

—*Edgar Allen Poe*

How do I stay inspired?

I am inspired by beauty. Whether it is in nature, in people, music, art, dance, theater, food—you name it, it's inspiring. I surround myself with beautiful things in my home environment. I have friends who are beautiful inside and out. The food that I eat is living and no harm is done to animals or myself when I eat it. With beauty surrounding me constantly, I am always inspired.

I am inspired by creativity. Artists, musicians, singers, poets, dancers, performers, and creators of all types inspire me. When I see an artist using colors in a unique way, I feel that inside me, and it sparks my creative juices in my own unique way as well.

I am inspired by mastery and success. When I see and experience people doing things I never thought possible, or even that I aspire to do but am not able to do yet, I am inspired. I love to grow, to progress and become better in all ways possible. When I see the potential of the human spirit, I am motivated to test my own potential as well. I invite you to do the same, while honoring yourself exactly where you are on your path!

I am inspired by happiness and love. There are unhappy people everywhere, and to be around them can really drag you down. I love to surround myself with others who are leading happy, successful, and fulfilling lives. We can encourage each other and be sources of positive reinforcement and strength. I empathize with those who are moving through challenges, as I have done so many times, but in the end I am most inspired by those who can maintain a loving, positive attitude despite what their circumstances may be at any given moment.

I am inspired by compassion. When I see people helping each other, offering their time, energy, and resources to a worthy cause to benefit the greater good of Earth or humanity, I am touched and moved. It deepens my commitment to my path and asks me to question whether I could be doing more for others than I am right now. I invite you to explore the same inquiry.

I am inspired by stories of transformation. Perhaps this is because my own path was challenging and I had to overcome many obstacles early in life to get to where I am. When I hear the stories people write to me about how yoga transformed their lives, how they are feeling so much better now, losing weight, sleeping better, overcoming heartbreak, depression, pain, illness, disease, or any number of other life transformation stories

I have had the blessing and privilege to experience, I am deeply touched. That is perhaps what motivates me more than all else. Your words touch my soul deeply, and it is the soul behind the words that I am feeling. That is the wealth. That is the rich reward that inspires me to continue offering my life in service with passion and joy!

Thank you for all that you are, all that you do, and all that you will do from now on. I honor your time and am so grateful to share this journey with you, even if it is over many miles and on paper through the transmission of these words. It is my heart, mind, and soul I am offering and sharing with you. My only request is that you apply the teachings in the Pranashama Yoga system and experience firsthand the life transformation I know is possible for you and everyone who follows even a few of these techniques.

I wish you joy and love at all times.
Om Sri Maha Laxshmiye Namaha.
May you be blessed with abundance, love, and beauty in the Holy name of the Divine.

Remember the Truth that You Are.

—*Lalla, eighth-century Kashmiri poet*

Poetic Inspiration by Dashama

Heart open.
Expanding energy in all directions.
Breath flowing
My mind's at peace—
As I create each moment with intention
and effortless ease.

Where do I go from here?

Outward and upward
Freely believing
Constantly conceiving
Raising my energy levels—
Reaching inside
Arresting my devils.

Breaking the bonds
That were holding me captive
I know that I came here
To live and let live.
To grow and evolve
And bring glory to God.
In my solemn appreciation
I offer my *prasad*
Up to the Creator
To show and give thanks
Purify my soul
At the serene riverbanks.

I'll cleanse my distractions
And purify my mind
Open my heart up

Pure love I will find.
No more illusions
No detours
No lies.
I'm seeking the truth now
There is no disguise
That can hide from me
The love that I seek . . .
That I am . . .
That you are . . .
The illusion is weak.

I've crushed it
And burned it
And cast it aside.
I know my pure essence
Grows stronger inside.

With each breath I take
And every action I make
I create a new world
Giving more than I take.
Brings joy to my soul
And peace to my heart
I see how beautiful
I can play my part—
And contribute to an awakening
By sharing the message loud and clear
Each moment that I'm breathing
I'm so grateful to be here.

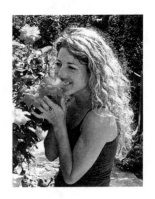

APPENDIX A

Self-Assessments

1. Self-assessment: Chakra Quiz/Where am I right now?

Please note: It is essential that you be completely open and honest with yourself in all of these assessments. Remember that no one is judging you, and you will only be hurting yourself and prolonging the attainment of your goals if you exaggerate or fudge the truth.

The following assessment will help you see if you are out of balance in any of your major energy centers, also know as chakras.

Please describe your attitude in the following categories in three words or less:

Mental Clarity _____

Physical Health _____

Spiritual Connectedness _____

Emotions _____

Take the following Chakra Personality Test (write Y or N to the left of the number):

I generally feel in harmony with the universe.

My intuition is quite well developed.

I express myself well in words.

I feel emotionally connected with other people.

I follow my gut instincts.

I am full of vitality and *joie de vivre*.

I love to be in movement and feel my own body.

It is easy for me to meditate and find inner peace.

I have good concentration.

I feel socially confident.

I am deeply afraid of loneliness.

Eating is one of the great pleasures of life.

I know how to enjoy life.

I almost never worry.

I find it difficult to take the world seriously.

I often think about the world and life.

I can easily put my thoughts into words.

Love is the most important thing in the world.

I am at peace within myself and not easily thrown off center.

I am a very passionate person.

I feel a deep connection with nature.

My soul's home does not lie in this world.

I have intense, color-filled dreams.

I have many different interests.

I have the desire to express myself artistically.

I experience feelings mostly in my body.

Sex is very important to me.

I have a lot of confidence in life and the future.

If you answer NO to any one of these items, you should look deeper into that aspect of yourself. If you have an area that is weaker than another, it is an opportunity for you to release old mental patterns that are keeping you stuck and embrace new thought forms that will raise your life to the next level in an upward-moving direction.

This is a very exciting opportunity and time for you! Be joyful for the process and honest in your evaluations.

By doing assessments like the one above, you are able to see yourself from an observer perspective and notice where you are experiencing imbalances. In this way, you can work on the weak or neglected areas and raise them to be in harmony with the other areas of your life. Remember that no one is perfect, but we are all striving to live in harmony and balance within ourselves, with the world around us, and with the universe. You will find tools and techniques in this book to utilize to bring your life into balance and then into an expanding state of continual evolution.

Additionally, answer the following questionnaire to establish your current goals and areas you need to work on.

My most frequently recurring thought about my life or myself is that I wish I were _____.

The reason(s) I don't exercise, do yoga, spend time with nature, meditate as often as I would like is (are) because _____
_____.

When I look in the mirror I see a person who _____
_____.

The most self-defeating recurring thought in my mind is that I am not _____ enough.

When I have thirty minutes of free time, I usually spend it _____
_____.

I believe the universe is inherently positive/negative (circle one). And it is here to challenge me/support me (circle one). It leads me to my struggle/ultimate enlightenment (circle one).

I feel (one word) _____ about my health and physical appearance.

My current relationships (including my relationship to myself) are fulfilling/in need of some healing (circle one).

I never/rarely/usually/always (circle one) experience road rage or anger while driving in heavy traffic.

I enjoy/neutral/despise (circle one) preparing and cooking meals for myself and/or others.

The natural environment (trees, forest, oceans, lakes, mountains) excite and rejuvenate me/scare me (circle one).

I think the global environmental crisis is out of my control/we can all do a little to make a change (circle one).

In my free time, when I want to relax I watch TV, computer, video games, eat or talk on the phone/do yoga, meditate, exercise, sing, dance, or play (circle one).

You will notice that each of these questions is evaluative of your current thoughts and habits that are creating your life scenario at every moment. You may begin to see, as you follow this guidebook, that as soon as you shift your thought patterns to affirm what you want to see and experience in your life, your whole experience here will improve. When you send positive, affirmative messages to the universe, you begin to attract the things you want into your life. This is why it is so important to decide what you truly want FIRST. If you don't know what you want, you will be attracting all sorts of situations, circumstances, and events into your life that may or may not support your ultimate dreams and goals.

You must become laser-focused on what you want, and unwavering in your approach to getting it. This is how the masters rise to mastery. It is how leaders rise to positions of power. And it is how you will rise to emulate your sublime vision for your life experience as well.

2. Schedule Assessment: Finding the Time for Yourself

We all have the same twenty-four hours in our day. So why is it, you may wonder, that some people are manifesting these blessed lives of abundance and joy, and others are struggling just to make ends meet?

This is a wonderful question.

First of all, if you haven't seen the movie *The Secret* or read the book, you should do that immediately. The amazing thing about the message that book has to offer lies in its profound simplicity.

With each thought you are manifesting and creating everything in your reality. You are attracting, directly from the Source of all Sources, all that you consciously and subconsciously desire.

It truly matters not where you were born, what circumstances you were raised in, and who your parents are. This fact is being confirmed time and time again. People born in slums and poverty, who have experienced all of life's struggles and challenges, rise to be a blessing unto their communities and live the lives they envision. One key to the mastery of your life is forming a loving relationship toward time and time prioritization. Most people have various relationships to time. Take a moment to assess your current relationship to time.

Negative relationships to time:

Wasting time

Killing time

Filling time

Passing time

Losing time

Time is escaping me

Time is flying by

Positive Relationships to time:

Finding the time

Making or creating time

Embracing time

Saving time

Using time wisely

Investing time

Sharing time

Infinitely life-enhancing relationships with time:

Experiencing timelessness

Going beyond all space and time

Befriending the concept of time

Becoming one with the concept of time

Aligning with time's infinite intelligence to attract all good things

The stillness of timelessness exists only within you. If you wish to slow time down so you can experience the fullness of a moment, you must transcend the chaotic chatter of your own mind. This happens only through meditation and the practice of silence.

If you have a long list of goals and things to do, time management and prioritization is of the highest importance. Below you will find an example of a time management sheet you can use to get yourself on track and create time to use to accomplish your goals.

Day: Monday

(This is all based upon a fictional workday for a typical 9 to 5 job.)

7 a.m.—wake up, shower

7:30 a.m.—thirty minutes of yoga/meditation to jump-start your day; read a positive affirmation for the day

8 a.m.—healthy energizing breakfast or protein smoothie; pack your yoga or workout clothes, along with a healthy snack and lunch for the day

8:30 a.m.—leave the house to be at work by 9 a.m. (Be sure to bring some uplifting music to listen to on your commute. The sound frequency will stay with you throughout the day.)

9 a.m.—arrive at work with the attitude that today is going to run smoothly and efficiently!

Noon—lunch: eat something prepared from the night before or a healthy meal from the local organic deli or restaurant; take a fifteen-minute walk in a natural environment/park, or sit by a body of water to recharge your spirit.

1 p.m.—arrive back at work recharged and ready for the afternoon of work productivity and efficiency.

5 p.m.—prepare to leave work and go to the gym, yoga studio, park, or beach to unwind from the day. This is one of the most essential aspects of your day. If you choose to skip this step, your evening will be far less enjoyable and you will allow energy to get stuck inside you that is begging to be released. This often leads to relationship challenges and arguments, etc.

7 p.m.—prepare or order a healthy dinner (some food choice ideas are included in Appendix D, "Introduction to the Three-Stage Energy Diet").

8 p.m.—read a book that will enhance or enrich your mind, body, spirit, or emotions. Additionally, this is a great time to study a new skill or trade that is more in alignment with your highest vision for your life, if you are not currently full-time working the fulfilling career of your dreams.

10 p.m.—write your goals and to-do list for the next day.

11 p.m.—do five minutes of stretching and five minutes of silent reflective visualization. Look back over the day to see what blessings you were graced with, and what challenges you faced and overcame. Be grateful for the gift of life to continue another day. Drift off into a blissful, relaxed dream world.

You will notice in a schedule like this that I have offered you several opportunities to stop, breathe, stretch, get in touch with yourself and how you are feeling, invoke feelings of gratitude in your heart, and work on yourself.

This may all sound ideal, and perhaps you are thinking, "Dashama, this is easy for you to say, but I have kids and responsibilities beyond just myself. I don't have the luxury to stop at yoga class after work; I must pick up the kids, or grocery shop, etc."

I'm here to say, "You create your reality." If you have kids, pets, responsibilities beyond just yourself, you are among a huge portion of the population. That is why it is even more important for you to prioritize your schedule and your time.

Ideally, you could have the schedule I have created for you above, but if it is impossible right now, you need to simply start somewhere and do what you can. And be a little selfish in the beginning. Many parents I meet selflessly sacrifice their entire health and happiness to be the chauffeur, maid, nanny, cheerleader, traveling soccer parent, etc. This is all wonderful, but if you neglect yourself, you will never be the parent you would be if you gave some of that time and attention to yourself. And when you do, you will see the miracle of life unfold! You will begin to notice how your children actually can do things for themselves; they will appreciate your presence at their games and activities even more; and your newfound radiance and positivity will spill forth onto them. Their lives will be enhanced by your choice to honor your own personal needs and desires.

A wise friend of mine, mother of four, grandmother of two, commented recently, "If everyone in the world just took care of themselves, we could see a lot more joy and peace." And this is absolutely true. We see many people trying to take care of their spouse, their children, their parents, their friends, lovers, co-workers, etc., and neglecting their own needs as a result of this. Perhaps it is out of avoidance of taking care of the self. Somehow it seems easier to fuss over others, and we have adopted subconscious belief systems that say we are selfish if we redirect that time and attention to our own lives. We may have learned this from our parents, who fussed over others and us just as much. It is proven that we model those who surround us growing up. It is our job to undo the family, societal, and social conditioning and reprogram ourselves to become balanced, abundant, Divine Creations deeply connected to the Source at all times.

This is a tall order. It may take some time. Be prepared—life is a journey. Each moment will be a test and a blessing.

Open your eyes and your heart to embrace every aspect of life in all of its richness. You will be rewarded for your dedication and commitment to excellence and the pursuit of your dreams.

Your turn!

Create your schedule now, making the effort to include activities that will bring you closer to your ideal vision of your life. Include relaxation, exercise, learning new hobbies, taking classes, spending time with friends and loved ones, meditation or inner reflection, journaling, reading, etc.

	Monday	Tuesday	Wednesday	Thursday	Friday	Saturday	Sunday
8 AM –							
9 AM –							
10 AM –							
11 AM –							
Noon –							
1 PM –							
2 PM –							
3 PM –							
4 PM –							
5 PM –							
6 PM –							
7 PM –							
8 PM –							

Be sure to leave some blocks of time open for spontaneous events and opportunities that may arise. This should be fun and will help you feel more in control and organized with your time. Remember that it is your life that you are sculpting, and the clay is malleable, not set in stone. This schedule can change and fluctuate just as your life does.

APPENDIX B

Chakras, Mantras, and the Power of Chanting

Understanding that yoga was created more than five thousand years ago as a science and complete system to balance and unify the individual self with the Universal Self, you will benefit profoundly by incorporating some techniques into your daily lifestyle. Following are some yogic exercises that can balance and open your energy centers/chakras and lead to your ultimate and highest experience in this life:

- **First Chakra:** *Physicality and Root.* Hamstring and other lower-body stretching poses: forward-bend variations, lunges, warrior poses, ground/mat sequences, as well as bridge pose, among others.
- **Second Chakra:** *Emotional Center.* Butterfly, wide-leg forward bending, inner thigh and hip-stretching poses like double warrior, lotus variations, camel pose variations, and bridge pose variations.
- **Third Chakra:** *Power Center.* Core-strengthening poses like boat pose, crow pose, and other arm balances that require strength from the core, balance core sequences, and variations of plank pose, to name a few.
- **Fourth Chakra:** *Heart Center.* Back-bending poses like full wheel, camel, *anahatasana* (heart to the earth pose), shoulder-stretching poses like eagle arms, reverse *namaste*, bow pose, and table, as well as arm-binding positions for more advanced practitioners.
- **Fifth Chakra:** *Throat Center.* Neck and shoulder stretching poses like fish, shoulder stand, plow, locust, rabbit, lion's breath, and

other exercises like chanting that will create resonant vibration into the throat center and release blocked energy.

- **Sixth Chakra:** Meditation and visualization are the best yoga practices to balance and open the sixth Chakra/Third Eye. In addition, eye exercises can help strengthen the pineal gland, and Tratak candle gazing can stimulate it as well.
- **Seventh Chakra:** Crown/Gate to God. Head stand and other inversions where the head is touching the earth, to release tension and stimulate and unblock energy from the crown of the head. Meditation, chanting, and visualization also help balance and open the crown chakra and increase your feeling of connectedness to the omnipotent presence of the Supreme Source that is within and all around—always—everything in existence.

Chanting and Working with Mantras

1. Aum
The Primal Shabda

Om, pronounced "Aum," is an affirmation of the Divine Presence that is the universe and is similar to the Hebrew "Amen." There are many ways of chanting Aum, but this is an approach that will initiate you as a Shabda Yogi, one who pursues the path of sound toward wholeness and higher states of consciousness.

2. Lokah Samastah
A Chant for Wholeness

Lokah samastah sukhino bhavantu.
May this world be established with a sense of well-being and happiness.

3. Gayatri
Being Illuminated by Sacred Sound
Om bhur bhuvas svaha
Thath savithur varaynyam
Bhargo dheyvasya dhimahih
Dhyoyonah pratchodhay-yath

We worship the word (*shabda*) that is present in the Earth, the heavens, and that which is beyond. By meditating on this glorious power that gives us life, we ask that our minds and hearts be illuminated.

4. Om Namah Shivaya

Om Namah Shivaya, Namah Shivaya, Nama Shiva
I bow to Lord Shiva, the peaceful one who is the embodiment of all that is caused by the universe.

5. Bija Mantras
Seed Mantras
In the "seed" (*bija*) mantras each seed is conceived of as the sound-form of a particular Hindu deity, and each deity is in turn a particular aspect of the Absolute (Brahman). It's said that just as a great tree resides within the seed, so does a god or goddess reside in each *bija*. When we chant the *bijas*, we identify each syllable with the divine energy they represent.

Sound	Pronunciation	Awareness
Lam	Curve the tip of your tongue up and back, and place it on the rear section of the upper palate to pronounce a sound like the word *lum* without the initial *a*.	Base of the spine
Vam	Place the upper set of teeth on the inner section of your lower lip and begin with a breathy consonant to imitate the sound of a fast car. Pronounce the *mantra* like "*fvam*."	Genitals
Ram	Place the tip of your tongue on the roof of the front section of the upper palate, roll the *r* as in Spanish, and pronounce the *mantra* like the first part of the word "rumble."	Abdomen
Yam	Inhale audibly through your mouth, and pronounce the word *hum* (as in humming); allow the breath to extend beyond the resolution of the consonant.	Solar Plexus and Heart Area
Ham	Inhale noiselessly through your mouth, and pronounce the sound like the word *yum* (as in yummy); allow the sound along with your breath to fill your mouth and throat cavity.	Throat
Om	Inhale audibly through your nostrils, and direct the stream of air to the point between your eyebrows. Pronounce the sound along with your exhalation as a subtly audible whisper, allowing the sound and breath to resonate in the cranial area.	Point between the Eyebrows

This is a must. Most people are a little hesitant about this aspect of yoga. It seems strange, and if you don't know the inherent benefits that come from the practice, you will not be inspired or motivated to begin or try it. So, allow me to share some insight.

First, we all know that thoughts and words are creative. They attract everything into your life. Second, chanting is one of the most healing and transformative practices that yoga has gifted us with. Actually, almost all cultures throughout the world use chanting or sound vibration healing in some way or another. It doesn't have to be esoteric or weird. You don't have to be a monk or Hindu. Similar to singing, **you are simply allowing your body to become an instrument, like a flute or a drum, for sound and vibration to move through.**

The human body is more than 70 percent water, with most of the rest being various textured matter like bones, tissue, muscles, and fat. The sound vibration that comes from chanting works on a physical and energetic level to heal, balance, and clear you of blockages, imbalances, and dis-ease. This is fundamental and profound, and not to be brushed off or taken lightly. For this reason, I highly recommend working with mantras and chanting. I do it all the time. The best way to get started is to work with the seed sound of all creation, OM. In Tantra Yoga, there is a mantra, called a bija mantra associated with each chakra, which will best balance and clear the energy in that center.

APPENDIX C

Organs and Corresponding Emotions

Organ	Emotion	Time	Element
Stomach	Disgust/Despair	7–9 a.m.	Earth
Spleen	Low Self-Esteem	9–11 a.m.	" " " "
Heart	Excessive Joy	11 a.m.–1 p.m.	Fire
Small Intestine	Vulnerable	1–3 p.m.	" " " "
Bladder	Irritation	3–5 p.m.	Water
Kidney	Fear	5–7 p.m.	" " " "
Circulation, Sex	Anxiety	7–9 p.m.	Fire
Triple Warmer	Confusion	9–11 p.m.	" " " "
Gall Bladder	Resentment	11 p.m.–1 a.m.	Wood
Liver	Anger	1–3 a.m.	" " " "
Lungs	Grief	3–5 a.m.	Metal
Large Intestine	Being Stuck	5–7 a.m.	" " " "

APPENDIX D

Introduction to the Three-Stage Energy Diet

Diet and nutrition are ambiguous areas for many people. It is difficult to break habits that were formed from childhood. If you were raised eating pork chops, French fries, and drinking Mountain Dew, it may be difficult for you to shift over to a healthy lifestyle right away. That is the reason I have created three stages to the plan. It is a process of integration in which you will evolve your taste buds and desires away from those primarily satisfied by comfort foods, fat, grease, salt, creaminess, and processed sugars.

Three-Stage Energy Diet Program

This is an exciting time. You will begin to see yourself and your life as a miracle as you start to see how everything you consume affects you either positively or negatively.

Stage 1: Eliminate Junk!

In the first stage you are encouraged to substitute whole grains and natural sugars for processed grains and starches. You learn the concept of "eat to live, don't live to eat." Moderation and discipline are introduced into your lifestyle. You begin to gain an appreciation for the colors of foods and what they have to offer.

Additionally, you will be introduced to the nutritional content of various foods that sustain and enhance your energy. You learn the basic and fundamental workings of the digestive system and begin to integrate food-combining strategies into your daily diet. You get acquainted and in touch with your internal system that may have been a stranger to you for your entire life. You replace harmful substances like high-fructose corn syrup and trans-fatty acids that have been linked to cancer, obesity, and heart disease. You finally make time for those eight to ten glasses of water you've known you needed to drink each day since childhood. The recipes and meal suggestions I offer will include some of what you are familiar with, to allow for easy transition to your new lifestyle. In this stage meat-eating is still common, and splurging on "unhealthy foods" is considered acceptable and even essential to the process. This is the perfect place for you to start if you are trying to lose a little weight and implement anti-aging principles. This is the diet that most personal trainers will be on and encouraging their clients to follow.

Stage 2: Integrate Superfoods

In the second stage you are introduced to the concept of cleansing and detoxification. You learn that, just like your car, you must maintain your body in the same way. Your internal organs are like the parts of your car. They must be cleansed and replenished regularly to keep the whole process running smoothly with no problems. When you begin to understand how the liver affects your energy, and how overconsuming alcohol and certain foods destroys the functionality of this vital organ, you start to make better consumption choices.

In this second stage, we begin to enjoy the taste of water and prefer it to other toxic beverages. We see its inherent purpose and value in our lives and look forward to its cleansing and renewing effects. We begin to enjoy the flavor of vegetables and look forward to trying new foods. When we eat out, we choose restaurants that offer the highest-quality foods, with a wide variety of health-enhancing options. We begin to enjoy home-cooked meals even more, since we are able to see the ingredients and feel comfort in knowing we are consuming only the highest life-enhancing foods to nourish the body.

This is a wonderful diet for people interested in attaining the highest state of health and balance, but who need to remain grounded in this material world. If you have obligations and family this will require some discipline, but it is manageable and highly rewarding on all levels.

Stage 3: Cleanse Your System

Stage 3 is the final level in this dietary process. This is when the magic happens. You see yourself as in control of yourself. And the more you know, the better you feel. The better you feel, the more you attract good things to yourself. In this way, you are consciously creating the life of your dreams. When we understand cleansing and detoxification, we can start to integrate the right foods into our diet that take care of this process for us naturally and continually.

We begin by eating at least one green-leafy colorful salad per day and consuming plenty of fresh fruits, seeds, nuts, raw and steamed vegetables, whole grains, and high-nutrient-density deliciousness. We crave foods that are alive and life-enhancing. We feel revitalized by our meals and snacks. We become very sensitive to our bodies, so we can detect when we are out of harmony immediately and implement specific strategies to rebalance ourselves. We consume moderately, and when we are consuming we focus completely on the process of chewing, swallowing, absorption, digestion, and elimination.

We see each meal as a gift of nourishment and a blessing from the Divine. We give thanks for each bite every time. To each glass of water we offer a blessing, knowing that our bodies are composed of more than 70 percent water, and the quality of our life is dramatically enhanced and improved when we increase the frequency of the water we consume. The diet is wonderful for healers, spiritual teachers and leaders, and those people who spend a great deal of time each day either in meditation or spiritual *sadhana*. At times you may feel incredibly "high" and almost as if you could fly! This allows for a transformative state of consciousness, yet can at times feel a bit ungrounded. This can easily be remedied by consuming grounding foods, which have a high density and low water content, such as nuts, fish, eggs, and grains like quinoa and millet.

Optional:

Stage 4: Detoxify Your Internal Organs

This last, optional stage is for you if you are ready to really feel great in your body. We continue on the Detox diet from Stage 3, while incorporating herbal cleanses into the program each day. You may be surprised to learn that your body should be cleansed and detoxified at least a few times per year. How often do you take your car in for an oil change?

You should be cleansing your internal organs and systems at least as often. There are herbal, natural, and safe cleanses available in every health and nutrition store in the world. The major cleanses that I recommend include: Colon, digestive organs, liver, kidney, parasites, and mercury/heavy metal programs.

Wait a minute! You may say: I certainly don't have any parasites or heavy metals in my body! And to that I reply: Most people do, and you are not alone.

In the world that we have created for ourselves here on planet Earth, everything is different than it was a hundred years ago. The food and water we drink may contain heavy metals and other non-essential trace elements. These accumulate in your body just like plaque builds up on your teeth if you don't brush them. That leads to decay, deterioration, sickness, and dis-ease.

You don't have to FEEL sick to BE sick or need a cleanse. In fact, you should get in the habit of doing it before any symptoms arise for you, as an effort toward illness prevention and preservation of your overall health and well-being. I look at it like health insurance. If you keep your body and internal systems clean and healthy, they won't be a breeding ground for disease and sickness. This means your likelihood of ending up with a chronic or terminal illness will be dramatically decreased. This will create a higher quality of life for you and for those who love you. This is key. We don't want to be a burden upon those who care about us (neither their hearts nor wallets), and one key to this is to keep ourselves healthy!

Tips

Eat small meals frequently instead of large meals a few times throughout each day. You may have heard this before, and you're going to hear it from me too. The reason is: it works, and if you are still not following these rules, you will continue to see the same results you've been getting in the attainment of your health goals. One definition of insanity is doing the same thing over and over and expecting a different result. You have to change some of your habitual patterns in order to see real, lasting, and measurable changes in your life.

Eat breakfast daily.

Eat moderately. What does this mean? It means eat until you are no longer hungry. It means don't eat until you're stuffed and can't fit another bite in your belly.

Most of the time we aren't even hungry when we start eating, so this rule is often lost from first bite. Before you begin eating, ask yourself: "Am I hungry?" If yes, how hungry? If you're only a little hungry, only eat a little bit. And even if you are very hungry, you should still not consume massive amounts of food. It takes your body much too long and takes too much energy to digest overconsumption. Medically speaking, overconsumption is directly correlated to many of the life-threatening health concerns of our time. It has been linked to everything from obesity to heart disease, cancer, stroke, and organ failure.

It is mentally, physically, spiritually, financially, and emotionally drain-ing. On the basic and immediately effective levels, oftentimes it creates the desire for a nap. This is because the body needs time and energy to perform the miracle of digestion, with the assistance of digestive enzymes and gastric juices. You can help your body do its job more efficiently by consuming moderately and ingesting additional pro-biotic enzymes, as well as chewing each bite until the food becomes soft and almost liquefied. The digestion process does begin in the mouth, and if we skip this step and swallow our food only partially chewed, we create more work for our digestive system and this often leads to indigestion and the resultant intestinal gases.

Get on a regular and continual eating schedule that supports your needs and fits into your lifestyle. It may take a bit of preparation to begin, and to have the best foods available for snacking and meals. Addi-tionally, you will feel like you're eating too much at first if you are used to the traditional three-square-meals-a-day approach. Most people these days aren't even following the traditional meal schedule. Eating has become very imbalanced and erratic. The concept of community and family unity has been lost in much of our society. It is ideal to eat with family, friends, and loved ones when we can. This maintains a sense of community and connectedness that was and should still be an integral aspect to the balance and harmony we experience in our lives.

Example eating schedule: 4–5 small meals/3–4 hours apart: 8 a.m., 11:30 a.m., 3 p.m., 6:30 p.m. OR 7 a.m., 10:30 a.m., 2 p.m., 5 p.m., 8 p.m. When you eat in this way, you allow your body to burn the "fuel" quickly and efficiently and you never allow your "internal fur-nace" to grow cold. It is important that you consume the right foods during these small meals as well. This is the key to maintaining a healthy metabolism and to losing excess fat.

For Fat and Weight Loss:

Follow the three stages of the Energy Diet plan. This will ensure that your weight loss will not only be gradual, which is the healthiest way to lose weight, but will be permanent. This is due to the fact that your new consumption habits will be a reflection of your new lifestyle and not part of a fad diet or weight loss plan. When you begin to clean up your consumption and become more conscious in all aspects of your life, you will see the weight melting off you.

You won't need to get on a scale ever again, since you will be able to see how much weight you have lost when you look at yourself in the mirror!

Organic Foods

It is best to consume foods labeled organic whenever possible. Organic foods are grown in nutrient-dense soil without the use of pesticides and other insect-killing poisons. These foods are not genetically modified either. Many foods that are sold in the stores today have been genetically modified in some way or another. Although the process of genetic modification has not been around long enough for extensive studies to be conducted, there are negative repercussions to consuming these foods. Foods that have had their genes altered tend to have longer shelf lives, while at the same time having a reduced nutrient content.

There are even some types of vegetables and fruits that have been genetically modified to be insect-repellent. Thus the beautiful, red, plump, juicy-looking tomato that we see in the produce section has the ability to kill various insects when they take a bite from it. Just imagine what this "product" is able to do to our bodies!

Additionally, if you choose to eat meat, try to eat meat that has been raised on an organic farm, fed with nutrient-dense grains and grasses. Most of the meats sold in the grocery stores have come from animals raised on factory farms that were fed hormones and steroids to make them grow faster and larger to gain greater profits for the meat industry. Still others are being injected with antibiotics to sustain the animals' lives despite their diseases and illnesses. There have been studies conducted that link human consumption of these hormones, etc., to various types of cancer and other life-threatening diseases.

If you wish to read more about the evolution of our food in America, I strongly suggest you read the book *The Food Revolution* by John Robbins.* It is a very well written and detailed account of our current dietary state and where our society is heading if we continue in the direction we have been thus far.

The physical body and the material aspect of your life are complex and could encompass volumes and novels. This information is not meant in any way to be finite or conclusive. Your body and physicality are very important and I encourage you to become interested in exploring ever deeper into this aspect of your existence.

Food Revolution: How Your Diet Can Help Save Your Life and Our World (San Francisco: Conari, 2010).

Eight Limbs of Yoga

Below are the Eight Limbs of the Ashtanga Yoga Path as outlined by Patanjali, grandfather of modern-day yogic science.

Yamas is your attitude toward others and the world around you.

There are five *yamas*:

Ahimsa or non-violence. This *yama* is not limited to not doing harm to others in thought and in deed, it also refers to practicing acts of kindness to other creatures and to one's own self.

Satya or truthfulness. *Satya* is the *yama* that is about living a truthful life without doing harm to others. To practice *satya*, one must think before he speaks and consider the consequence of his action. If the truth could harm others, it might be better to keep silent.

Asteya or non-stealing. This *yama* is not only concerned about the avoidance of stealing material objects but also the stealing of others' ideas and forms of possession. Using power for selfish motives or telling someone else about confidential information you had been entrusted with is against *asteya*.

Bramacharya or non-lust. *Bramacharya* means to move toward the essential truth or to achieve self-control, abstinence, or moderation, especially regarding sexual activity. It is about not giving in to our ego's excessive desires or taking nothing in excess.

Aparigraha or non-possessiveness. This *yama* is about living a life free from greed or taking only what is necessary and not taking advantage of someone or a situation. It is about using our powers correctly and appropriately and not exploiting others.

Niyama is how you treat yourself or your attitude toward yourself.

Following are the five Niyamas:

1. **Sauca or cleanliness.** This niyama is concerned with both the outer and inner cleanliness. The practice of pranayama, asanas, and yogic cleansing to detoxify and cleanse the physical body is necessary to achieve inner cleanliness. The mind must also be kept clean or pure. Outer cleanliness, on the other hand, means to keep a clean environment or surroundings.

2. **Santosha or contentment.** Santosha involves practicing humility and modesty, and finding contentment with what you have and who you are.

3. **Tapas or austerity.** This niyama refers to keeping the body in good condition. Tapas is practiced through disciplining the body, speech, and mind, such as eating only when hungry and maintaining a good posture.

4. **Svadhyaya or study of the sacred text and of one's self.** This involves studying one's self through self-inquiry, self-examination, and other things that can help you get to know yourself better. As your knowledge about yourself grows deeper, so does your connection to the higher power and your union with all things.

5. **Isvarapranidhana or living with an awareness of the Divine.** This niyama encourages us to let go of our false sense of control and to connect to the Divine or that which gives us the sense of wholeness and sacredness.

Asanas or Physical Poses

The asanas are designed to free our mind and body from tension and stress. This practice relaxes, rejuvenates, and energizes the body and aims to bring the body and the mind into a harmonious union. Asanas should be done with comfort, ease, alertness, and steadiness, achieving a balance between ease and effort.

Pranayama or Breathing Exercises

Pranayama is the control of breath. The breath is regulated and controlled through the practice of breathing exercises. The duration of inhalation, retention, and exhalation of breath is regulated with the aim of strengthening and cleansing the nervous system and increasing a person's source of life energy. *Pranayama* practice also makes the mind calmer and more focused.

Pratyahara or Withdrawal of the Senses

This occurs during meditation, *pranayama*, or *asana* wherein you are so focused and immersed in your yoga, meditation, or breathing practice that you become unaware of outside situations. Your focus moves inward and you are no longer distracted by outside events.

Dharana or Concentration

Dharana is training the mind to focus without any distraction. To achieve this, you can focus your mind on one object at a time. This can also serve as a preparation for meditation.

Dhyana or Meditation

Meditation is the practice by which there is constant observation of the mind. It means focusing the mind on one point, stilling the mind in order to perceive the Self. It is an uninterrupted flow of concentration aimed to heighten one's awareness and oneness with the universe. It is also an important tool to achieve mental clarity and health.

Samadhi or Enlightenment

This is the ultimate goal of the Eight Limbs of Yoga. It is characterized by the state of ecstasy and the feeling that you and the universe are one. It is a state of peace and completion, awareness and compassion with detachment.

APPENDIX F

Finding a Teacher

For years, people have come to me to help them relieve some stress from their lives. The strain and burden of work, family, finances, and illness all build up in the body. This often goes on for years unaddressed, contributing to the rapid decay of physical health. Muscles become so tight and knotted it feels like they are made of iron rods and steel bolts. Heartbeats and breathing are completely erratic and unsupportive to the nervous system. Blood circulation begins to falter and coagulate. Veins become broken and visible through the skin. Strokes and heart palpitations manifest. Migraine headaches and TMJ tension disorders are commonplace these days. The list can go on and on.

How are you living under these conditions?

By the time a client comes to me, usually they are at the end of their rope. They have allowed the stress and tension to build up for so long that the repercussions are becoming severe, sometimes even debilitating. It takes a lot of strength and humility on the level of the ego to ask for help. Usually a person will contemplate starting a therapy of some sort for a while before they actually pick up the phone. I have had people tell me they saw my website a year ago and are just now ready to get started.

There are many reasons why people hesitate. If they only knew the best therapies available that were effective and cost-efficient, it may be a lot easier. Most of the time people just start searching online and asking their doctor or a few close friends for advice. What works? What might help? In this manual, I include the most effective therapies and suggestions I have known to be proven and time-tested. Everything I suggest to you I have utilized to heal my own life and the lives of my friends and clients throughout the years.

Keep in mind that everyone is unique. Your path is not identical to mine or anyone else's. It will benefit you most to try a variety of therapies to find the best path for yourself. The best path is always the one that brings you the most steady and consistent joy, most rapidly.

Since the purpose and ultimate goal in life is to be HAPPY, everything that puts you closer to that state of being is beneficial.

When deciding to improve your health, it is often necessary to hire a trainer, coach, or teacher to guide you on your path. These professionals are skilled in techniques and can offer tools that will dramatically enhance your healing process in a rapid way. Below is a list of healing therapies that I have come to know will help you on your path to living a life in harmony and balance with your ultimate vision.

As you review this list, you will naturally be drawn to certain items. Go with your initial instinct when moving forward with a therapy. And think of this as a fun and exciting new venture where you will be able to learn a lot about yourself on all levels. You will tap into the deepest levels of your being and discover the roots of your current behavior and lifestyle patterns. After making these discoveries, you can release them much more easily.

Physical Therapies

1. Yoga
2. Chakra therapy
3. A moderate lifestyle
4. Dietary evolution and conscious consumption
5. Fitness
6. Acupuncture
7. Thai Yoga bodywork
8. Liberation through dance and movement therapy
9. *Panchakarma*/detoxification
10. Massage therapy

Mental Therapies

1. Meditation
2. Hypnosis
3. NLP (Neuro-Linguistic Programming)
4. The Forum by Landmark Education or any such group therapy
5. Mantras
6. Affirmations
7. Observation of thoughts
8. Talk therapy and traditional counseling
9. Eradication of addictions, especially the intake of toxins such as alcohol, cigarettes, and drugs
10. Feng shui

Emotional Therapies and Spiritual/Energetic Therapy

1. Cord Cutting
2. Transformational Breathwork
3. Loving Relationship Training
4. Artistic and creative expression
5. Tantric energy work
6. Nature therapy
7. Reiki
8. Qigong and T'ai Chi
9. Karma Yoga
10. Chanting and singing

The ability to quantify your progress is very useful as you advance along on your path. For instance, if you could stand to lose a few pounds to improve your physical health, as you do improve in this area you will notice your self-esteem rising and your mental self-talk getting more positive and encouraging. In turn, your emotional well-being will be more balanced as you see the progress you are making, and your overall connectedness to your Higher Spiritual self will feel stronger and more rewarding. This is just one example of how this process works.

In Pranashama Yoga, all evolution is held in the highest regard. Any and all efforts you make toward the rebalancing and evolution of your life are acknowledged and worthy of praise and acknowledgement. Remember to reward yourself along the way for your small incremental progress, as well as for the large and notable successes. You will stay motivated and filled with enthusiasm as you progress if you have something to look forward to along the way. An example of this would be giving yourself a "free day" after your tenth yoga session, in which you are able to do anything you desire, or nothing at all! This type of reward will revive you to continue on. Small breaks always reaffirm the value and benefit of the therapy, as you will experience a noticeable difference between how you feel with it and without it. When you reach larger goals, like a paramount weight loss or a breakthrough in a relationship you were struggling with, give yourself a larger reward. Maybe buy a plane ticket to go somewhere you love to go. Spend time doing what you love and relish the joy and gratitude for reaching that next level in your highest evolution.

Blessings to you on your path.

Index

About the Author

Dashama Konah Gordon is a yoga teacher, author, performing artist, and inspirational speaker. She has practiced hatha yoga since childhood and is part of a rising generation of young celebrity instructors who incorporate life coaching skills in their yoga teaching. Gordon graduated from the Sivananda TTC (Teacher Training Course), one of the oldest and most widely recognized yoga certifications, established over 40 years ago by Swami Vishnudevananda. She has since trained with Shiva Rea in yoga and Mukti Michael Buck in Thai Yoga Bodywork. She holds a bachelors degree in Intercultural Communication and International Relations from Florida Atlantic University and presently travels the world sharing the gift of yoga and life transformation.

Gordon cofounded the 30 Day Yoga Challenge, a program for transforming people's lives, partnering with National Yoga Month (yoga-month.org) to bring yoga via video and the internet to those who have no access to local classes. The 30 Day Yoga Challenge program will be available as a downloadable app. She has starred in five yoga DVDs and plans to write more books on her personal approach to yoga. Current projects include developing her own Yoga Alliance-recognized teacher-training program, the Pranashama Yoga® School, and an internet TV reality show called *Transform Your Life with Dashama*.